THE TARZAN RULE

TIPS FOR A HEALTHY LIFE IN MEDICINE

Mamta Gautam, MD, FRCPC

THE TARZAN RULE:
TIPS FOR A HEALTHY LIFE IN MEDICINE
Mamta Gautam, MD, FRCPC

2011© Mamta Gautam
1-72 Queen Elizabeth Drive
Ottawa, ON Canada
K2P 1E4
(613) 729-3794
www.peakmd.ca

Published by:
Partner Publishing, Ottawa, ON, Canada
www.partnerpublishing.com
info@partnerpublishing.com

Cover and graphic design: Donald Lanouette
Editing: Karen Opas

Library and Archives Canada Cataloguing in Publication
Gautam, Mamta, 1961-

The Tarzan Rule: Tips for a Healthy Life in Medicine, Mamta Gautam

Includes bibliographical references.
ISBN: 978-0-9784701-7-3

1. Physicians-Pyschology 2. Physicians-Job Stress
3. Physicians-Mental health 4. Stress management

For my mother, Rama.
All I know about caring for others,
I learned from you.

Alan - this book would
never have been written
without you. Thank
you for your advice,
support, guidance and
encouragement over
the years.

Love,
Mamta

ACKNOWLEDGEMENTS

This book would never have been written without the amazing people at the *Medical Post*, an independent newspaper and information source for Canada's doctors. I shall always remain grateful to them for sharing my vision to promote Physician Health broadly, and their encouragement and support for the column, "Helping Hand," which I have written for over seven years, and which forms the basis of this book. Matt Borsellino was the *Medical Post* reporter who covered the very first conference on Physician Health at which I spoke, and became a key fixture at every similar conference for years after. He astutely recognized the value and increasing role that physician health would play in the future of medicine, and wrote about each and every innovation and development in this field, so physicians around the country could become aware of, and benefit from, them. Matt and I first spoke about the idea of the monthly column on issues related to Physician Health, and the idea took root. Matt connected me to Joe McAllister, one of the most capable and patient editors in the world. Joe helped with the name of the column, "Helping Hand," and guided, reminded, and edited me for years. I always looked forward to the annual lunch in Toronto with Matt and Joe, where we would chat about the column for a bit and then just get on with enjoying each other's company. Over the years, I have also greatly appreciated working with Colin Leslie, Rick Campbell, and David Hodges. A huge thank you to all of you.

I owe the title of this book entirely to Drs. Alan Buchanan and Anthony Sehon. They shared the concept of the Tarzan Rule with me after a presentation I gave at one of their Psychiatric Update for Family Physicians conferences. You will read more about it throughout the book, and realize why I felt that this concept embodied the theme of this book. I am overwhelmed by Alan and Tony's generosity of spirit in sharing and allowing me to use this idea. They are very special colleagues and mentors to me.

Reviewing all the columns I had written over the years, Steve Wharry suggested that I put them together into a book. Great idea, Steve—thanks. Putting a book together takes expertise, knowledge, patience, and thought. Luckily, I had all of these attributes in Karen Opas and Donald Lanouette of Partner Publishing, who led the editing, cover design, and publishing process. Thank you for your help and guidance in bringing this book to life.

I want to thank my colleagues in the area of Physician Health across Canada and around the world who work each day to assist other physicians in regaining and maintaining their health so they can continue to take care of others. I also want to thank the colleagues who trust us to help them through difficult times.

My family and friends keep me healthy and happy. My husband, Kiran, is a never-ending source of love, gentleness, and grace. Nikesh, Shaun, and Neal, my three sons, fill me with pride, and remind me of the need to laugh and live each day fully. My mother continues to inspire me and remind me of what I have achieved, and encourage me to constantly expand my vision of Physician Health. My sisters, Rita, Vinita, Alka, and Monica laugh and cry with me as required. I learn something from each of my nieces and nephews every time I see them. My friends are always there to nurture and reenergize me, and celebrate all of life's moments. I look forward to a million more special moments with each of you.

TABLE OF CONTENTS

•

TABLE OF CONTENTS

•

TABLE OF CONTENTS

SECTION SEVEN
MAINTAINING YOUR PEAK PERFORMANCE:
RESILIENCY IN MEDICINE

BIBLIOGRAPHY

ABOUT THE AUTHOR

●

THE TARZAN RULE

TIPS FOR A HEALTHY LIFE IN MEDICINE

Mamta Gautam, MD, FRCPC

THE TARZAN RULE:
TIPS FOR A HEALTHY LIFE IN MEDICINE
Mamta Gautam, MD, FRCPC, MOT

2011© Mamta Gautam
1-72 Queen Elizabeth Drive
Ottawa, ON Canada
K2P 1E4
(613) 729-3794
www.peakmd.ca

Published by:
Partner Publishing, Ottawa, ON, Canada
www.partnerpublishing.com
info@partnerpublishing.com

Cover and graphic design: Donald Lanouette
Editing: Karen Opas

Library and Archives Canada Cataloguing in Publication
Gautam, Mamta, 1961-

The Tarzan Rule: Tips for a Healthy Life in Medicine, Mamta Gautam

Includes bibliographical references.
ISBN: 978-0-9784701-7-3

1. Physicians-Pyschology 2. Physicians-Job Stress
3. Physicians-Mental health 4. Stress management

For my mother, Rama.
All I know about caring for others,
I learned from you.

ACKNOWLEDGEMENTS

This book would never have been written without the amazing people at the *Medical Post*, an independent newspaper and information source for Canada's doctors. I shall always remain grateful to them for sharing my vision to promote Physician Health broadly, and their encouragement and support for the column, "Helping Hand," which I have written for over seven years, and which forms the basis of this book. Matt Borsellino was the *Medical Post* reporter who covered the very first conference on Physician Health at which I spoke, and became a key fixture at every similar conference for years after. He astutely recognized the value and increasing role that physician health would play in the future of medicine, and wrote about each and every innovation and development in this field, so physicians around the country could become aware of, and benefit from, them. Matt and I first spoke about the idea of the monthly column on issues related to Physician Health, and the idea took root. Matt connected me to Joe McAllister, one of the most capable and patient editors in the world. Joe helped with the name of the column, "Helping Hand," and guided, reminded, and edited me for years. I always looked forward to the annual lunch in Toronto with Matt and Joe, where we would chat about the column for a bit and then just get on with enjoying each other's company. Over the years, I have also greatly appreciated working with Colin Leslie, Rick Campbell, and David Hodges. A huge thank you to all of you.

I owe the title of this book entirely to Drs. Alan Buchanan and Anthony Sehon. They shared the concept of the Tarzan Rule with me after a presentation I gave at one of their Psychiatric Update for Family Physicians conferences. You will read more about it throughout the book, and realize why I felt that this concept embodied the theme of this book. I am overwhelmed by Alan and Tony's generosity of spirit in sharing and allowing me to use this idea. They are very special colleagues and mentors to me.

Reviewing all the columns I had written over the years, Steve Wharry suggested that I put them together into a book. Great idea, Steve—thanks. Putting a book together takes expertise, knowledge, patience, and thought. Luckily, I had all of these attributes in Karen Opas and Donald Lanouette of Partner Publishing, who led the editing, cover design, and publishing process. Thank you for your help and guidance in bringing this book to life.

I want to thank my colleagues in the area of Physician Health across Canada and around the world who work each day to assist other physicians in regaining and maintaining their health so they can continue to take care of others. I also want to thank the colleagues who trust us to help them through difficult times.

My family and friends keep me healthy and happy. My husband, Kiran, is a never-ending source of love, gentleness, and grace. Nikesh, Shaun, and Neal, my three sons, fill me with pride, and remind me of the need to laugh and live each day fully. My mother continues to inspire me and remind me of what I have achieved, and encourage me to constantly expand my vision of Physician Health. My sisters, Rita, Vinita, Alka, and Monica laugh and cry with me as required. I learn something from each of my nieces and nephews every time I see them. My friends are always there to nurture and reenergize me, and celebrate all of life's moments. I look forward to a million more special moments with each of you.

TABLE OF CONTENTS

•

TABLE OF CONTENTS

•

TABLE OF CONTENTS

SECTION SEVEN
MAINTAINING YOUR PEAK PERFORMANCE:
RESILIENCY IN MEDICINE

BIBLIOGRAPHY

ABOUT THE AUTHOR

•

SECTION ONE

MEDICINE IS AN ENDURANCE SPORT: INTRODUCTION

Going Where Life Takes You

It has been over twenty years since I first set up my private practice in Psychiatry. I stop to reflect on where I started out, where I thought I would go, and where I am now. What an interesting ride!

The focus of my work has been Physician Health, at clinical, educational, administrative, and research levels. A Child Psychiatrist by training, I got into this area of specialty by pure serendipity.

My oldest son was born in my last year of residency, and the twins were born the following year in my first year of fellowship. I prepared to finish my training, expecting to enjoy a career as a child psychiatrist in the hospital setting. I met with my department chair to see how I could manage this with the three young children, hoping to explore options about flexible workload, modified schedule, or reduced call with reduced pay. The answer was swift and clear; "You will need to do what everyone else is doing; take it or leave it." After much consideration, I decided to leave and set up a private practice that would also allow me to spend time with my young family.

A few months later, I received a call from a dear friend on a Friday evening. She was that year's National President of the Federation for Medical Women (FMWC), and was hosting the Annual Scientific meeting. She had called to tell me that the speaker scheduled for 8 a.m. the following morning had become ill and asked if I could fill in. I agreed to help out a friend, sorted out daycare, and gave a seminar on Depression. At the end of this talk, three colleagues came up to speak to me separately. I still remember their similar comments "I felt as if you were talking about me...That's my story you were telling...I never realized that's what was happening to me." Then they continued, "You are not weird like I thought psychiatrists were. Will you take me on as a patient?" They were my first three physician patients, and within a year, through word of mouth, my practice was limited to caring for colleagues. This remained as the focus of my practice for twenty years. In addition to my clinical practice, I have worked to raise awareness of physician health issues, reduce stigma that can be a barrier to receiving help, deliver educational presentations and workshops, and collaborate with caring colleagues to create wellness programs and therapeutic networks to assist physicians in need.

I know that stress in medicine is the norm. There are multiple demands on us, especially with diminishing resources and the restructuring of health care. We try to be all things to all people. As a full-time clinician and educator, mother of three sons, and the wife of a physician, I have often experienced these stressors firsthand. None of my friends, colleagues, and patients are immune to them, either.

During my year as President of the Ontario Psychiatric Association, I set the presidential theme to highlight physician health issues. At a session in the Annual Scientific Meeting, we spoke about the role of media in influencing attitudes and public perceptions about mental illness, and creating and perpetuating stigma and discrimination. There was a reporter in attendance from the *Medical Post* who spoke up and suggested that the media can also play a positive role to reduce stigma and challenged us to explore ways to do so.

As a result, I began to write "Helping Hand," a regular column in the *Medical Post* since 2004. This column's intent is to normalize physicians' need for a helping hand from time to time, to serve as a forum on Physician Health, and to allow physicians to ask such questions as needed. It was hoped that it would assist to promote physician health, to teach physicians essential self-care skills, and reinforce healthy preventive behaviour. It allowed colleagues to ask for advice or assistance in a safe and anonymous manner, and to benefit from each other's experiences.

It has been an amazing experience for me. I have connected with medical colleagues from all over the country, who write to me, share their stories, and allow me to spread their insight and experience so other colleagues can benefit. I have learned just how lucky we are in the physicians we have in this country. The medical profession is full of dedicated, passionate, hard-working, empathetic, credible professionals with integrity. I feel humbled to be a part of this profession.

This book is a compilation of a selection of edited *Medical Post* columns written over the years, with some attempt made to reorganize them around loose themes.

These stories build on the metaphor of the *IronDoc*, my last book, in which I introduce the IronDoc as a doctor who trains and paces to participate in an endurance event—medicine. Success throughout our career requires not just initial training to produce results, but ongoing training to attain and maintain peak performance. Through my company, PEAK MD, I work with physicians, health care leaders, and health care teams to cultivate and promote leadership resilience and ongoing wellbeing.

These stories are the ones that touched audiences the most—the columns that resulted in volumes of letters, emails, laughter, and tears. The last letter I received stated "That's my story you were telling," reminding me of what that first physician patient had told me twenty years ago. I have come full circle. I thought I was going to practice child psychiatry, and here I am with the privilege of caring for my physician colleagues. I have learned to listen to my heart, seize opportunities, and go where life takes me. While I did not set out to come here, somewhere, somehow, I have achieved exactly what I had started out to do.

SECTION TWO

CULTIVATING PEAK PERFORMANCE: ISSUES IN PHYSICIAN HEALTH

SECTION TWO

Why Do We Do This To Ourselves?

A female colleague had been practicing medicine for ten years. She was trying to do it all—be the best doctor she could be, be there for her spouse, be the model parent, coach her kid's soccer team, make sure the house was running smoothly. "I feel like I am trying to please everyone and, some days, end up feeling like I have pleased no one at all. Many of my colleagues are the same. Why do we do this to ourselves?"

Physicians are not all the same, but we do share many characteristics that make us try to do it all, and become more vulnerable to stress. These include:

Being conscientious, highly responsible –e.g., making one last round on the wards before heading home for the day, even though someone else is now on call

Perfectionist, attending to all details –e.g., taking a long time to write progress notes, sometimes putting them off because we think it will require a lot of time and effort, and ending up with a pile of paperwork to do. This also makes it hard to delegate and let others help, as we feel they will not do it to our standards.

Needing control – of ourselves and our environment. Often, we feel anxious if we feel out of control, and so struggle to maintain tight control to alleviate anxiety. This makes it hard to let go, and relax.

Need for approval – we try to please others constantly, wanting to be liked. Yet, we are not always comfortable with praise or approval, and so dismiss or negate it when received. This makes it hard for us to set limits and say "No."

Chronic self-doubts – we feel like "impostors," having fooled others into thinking we know what we are doing for now. We worry about being found out, about having our cover blown, and people realizing just how little we really know. This makes us continue to achieve and do more, thinking what we have done may not be good enough.

CULTIVATING PEAK PERFORMANCE

Ability to delay gratification – we put off doing things for ourselves, as there is always something more we can do for others. This is what allowed us to do well in university, medical school, and residency. We never reassess this, and assume that if we continue do this, we will get recognition and reward. Unfortunately, in medicine, this becomes the standard and is expected, not rewarded; it can lead to overwork and stress. Not only do we put things off for ourselves, we also make these choices for our family.

These traits are not negative. In fact, they are the very same traits that make us succeed in medicine. Medicine selects for these personality types. Our teaching, our training, and even our patients, reinforce this behaviour.

It helps to know that we do have these traits, and to recognize them when they are evident. Our challenge is going to be, after accepting and acknowledging them, to set limits to them. We need to know when we need to be like this, and when we do not, so we can learn to relax these high expectations of ourselves, and enjoy being "good enough."

Juggling Five Balls: Balancing Our Lives at Home & Work

My colleague was racing home at lunch to bake a birthday cake for her son. Her morning office was running late, but she really wanted to make that special cake herself, and get back in time for her afternoon patients.

There is so much to do, and we want to do our best for our patients and colleagues, our family and friends, and our self. Some days, we don't know if we're coming or going! How can we best balance all that we have to do?

First of all, it helps to take a deep breath, and know that we are not alone. Balancing our work and home lives is one of the biggest challenges physicians face, and unfortunately, one that our medical studies did not prepare us for. It is an issue for both male and female physicians, since the traditional family with the father working and a stay-at-home mother is no longer the norm, and both parents struggle to balance their lives. However, it remains true that the woman, regardless of whether she works outside of the home or not, retains the bulk of the responsibility for housework and childcare.

Balancing is all about making choices. As physicians, we are bright, interested, capable, and competent. There are a lot of things we like, we enjoy doing, and that we are good at. We cannot do them all, even though we would like to. Balancing is so hard for us because it requires that we choose from all of these possibilities, and choose to do some, and (here's the hard part), choose to not do others. The challenge is in giving up things we like, that we are good at doing, things that we want to do! As has been said, we can do everything we want, just not all at the same time.

The concept of Phases is crucial. We go through many phases in life—studying, medical school and residency, being single, newly married, setting up a practice, having young children, adolescents, empty nesters, retirement…This means that there is no one perfect solution; just a workable solution for the phase of life we happen to be in at present. This is reassuring, because it means that if we choose to give up something we really like, it is just for now; when we reach another phase, we can make a different choice and return to something we had to give up earlier.

To make these choices, we need to set priorities in life. These priorities need to include work, but must also take into account our personal responsibilities to our family, friends, and to ourselves. Let me remind you of the story about The Five Balls. Life is a juggling act, and you are juggling five balls—**work, home, family, friends, and self-care**—and doing your best to keep them all in the air. Remember that the work ball is the only rubber one; that if you drop it, it will bounce back up, even higher than before. The other four are much more fragile, and need extra care so they do not become damaged.

Above all else, take care of yourself first. Every time you get on an airplane, you are given the safety demonstration. You are told that if the oxygen pressure in the plane drops, you are to secure your own oxygen mask first, before you assist anyone traveling with you who may require help. This is because you are no good to anyone else if you have passed out! Use the oxygen mask as a metaphor in your daily life. When you are feeling stress from multiple demands, stop and take the time to "put your own mask on first," that is, meet a need of your own that will allow you to continue to meet the needs of others. This is not a luxury, or something you need to feel guilty about (the topic of guilt among physicians would take up its own chapter!)—see it as an "investment" in all of your other roles and responsibilities.

The Number One Cause of Stress: The Number One Solution

Stress is inherent in medicine. A certain amount of stress is positive, motivating, and enriching. Beyond this, it turns to distress, which is what most of us mean when we say stress.

Walking together to the parking lot at the end of rounds one day, a colleague shared with me. "I find being a doctor very stressful. There is so much asked of me, and I can never do it all. I am hearing a lot about stress and burnout. I am afraid that I might have it and not even know."

Knowing what to watch out for is crucial. There are some early warning signs of stress. These include:

Increases in physical problems and illnesses. This is when that cold is now going into its third week, and looking back, you realize that you have had many more colds in the past year than usual.

Increased problems with relationships, both at home and at work. There is more irritability, disagreements, and conflicts; people complain that lately all you seem to do is pick fights.

Increases in negative thoughts and feelings. You are feeling negative about people, activities, and things you used to like. You start to feel that you have little or no choice, are stuck, and are being acted upon.

Increases in bad habits. These can include doing things that are not good for us, such as overeating, overspending, and drinking too much. Alternatively, it can include *not* doing things that are good for us, such as exercising or talking with a friend.

Exhaustion. Many of us walk around with a huge amount of stress, but remain upright and cope (vertical stress). Exhaustion is when we are so overwhelmed, that we cannot even get up to do it again for another day (horizontal stress).

Burnout is chronic emotional stress. It is not a medical diagnosis; rather a description of this situation of overstress. It has three main stages, as described by Christina Maslach.

1. *Emotional exhaustion*. We feel that we have little left to give. For most physicians, their ability to function at work is the last to be affected. They get through their workday, but can do little else. They are drained, irritable, and just want to be left alone. If anyone asks anything else of them, they "bite their heads off."

2. *Depersonalization*. It becomes too hard to deal with others outside of work, and we cut ourselves off socially and avoid people. At work, we stop going to rounds and meetings. At home, we stop returning phone calls, cancel social plans, and prefer to be alone. We develop negative attitudes; we come to dislike people we used to enjoy spending time with.

3. *Reduced sense of personal accomplishment*. At this advanced stage, we feel worthless, unproductive, and may adopt a cynical and distant approach to patients and work. Many physicians start to question what they are achieving at work, and think about leaving medicine entirely.

When Canadian physicians were surveyed by the Canadian Medical Association in 2003, 45.7 % of physicians responding felt they were in advanced stages of burnout. While more recent surveys show that this number is declining, physicians will always remain at risk of burnout.

While burnout is not a psychiatric diagnosis, left unaddressed, it can lead to serious difficulties. Serious consequences of burnout can include:

- Impaired job performance.

- Increased risk of medical errors.

- Professional problems, such as complaints, lawsuits, loss of hospital privileges, restriction and loss of medical license.

- Changing jobs, reducing work hours.

- Difficulty with relationships, both at home and work.

- Physical illnesses.

- Substance abuse and addictions.

- Psychiatric Illnesses, including anxiety and depression.

- Suicide.

There is no single or easy way to deal with stress. Yet, the following is worth bearing in mind. All stress, regardless of the reason for it, is because, there is a sense of lacking control and choice; of feeling trapped and stuck in the particular situation. If feeling a lack of control is the main cause of stress, then the main solution is to challenge this perception and focus on what we do control.

Control is an illusion; the only thing we control is our self. Often, we are trying to control aspects of the situation outside of us, and so appropriately feel that we have no control. We need to focus back on our role—our thoughts, feelings, expectations, hopes, needs, strengths, weaknesses—and modify this to regain a sense of control and manage our stress.

Neighborhood Watch

A colleague expressed concerns about her office partner. Recently, he seemed less reliable than usual, and was cancelling commitments regularly. He would come into work late most days, and was often dishevelled. Last week, she smelled alcohol on his breath. She was not sure if or how to approach him about this.

That physician was lucky to have her as a colleague; she obviously cared about him. A key aspect of a healthy work environment is a situation in which people look after each other. The University of Ottawa's Faculty of Medicine Wellness Program encourages development of such a Neighborhood Watch, defining the workplace as a neighborhood where people look out for each other, and assist as needed.

Generally, the incidence of substance use by physicians is similar to the incidence in the general population. However, physicians tend to have a more severe problem, as their income can support greater use, and they have access to special and serious medications and drugs.

The best resource for such a situation is a Physician Health Program. These exist in some form in every Canadian province or territory. These programs can assist in connecting the physician to needed resources for intervention, assessment, and management, and in some provinces, provide ongoing monitoring and advocacy for the physician in recovery. The College does not need to be involved in any way as long as the physician meets the expectations of the monitoring program. To find out more, you can contact your provincial or territorial Physician Health Program (PHP), or the Canadian Medical Association's Centre for Physician Health and Well-being.

The first thing to do in such a situation is to document your colleague's concerning behaviours at work. Even small signs of difficulty are important, as this may indicate advanced addictive behaviour. Most physicians are able to cover problems at work, and so work is often the last arena of their life to be affected.

You can approach this colleague yourself, and tell him you are concerned about his health, and give specific details on what you have noticed that causes you concern. In addition to outlining concerns, you must also specify consequences that may occur if things do not improve, and resources that offer assistance. Sometimes, colleagues are relieved that someone has noticed, and can validate and support their need for help. They can then be encouraged to contact their family physician, and/or the provincial physician support program.

However, be prepared to have your colleague deny any problem or brush off your concerns. Only 20% of physicians with substance abuse/dependence will contact resources on their own behalf; and then, often only if there is a crisis resulting from this behaviour.

If you are concerned about the impairment of this physician's judgment, and his ability to practice medicine with skill and safety towards patients, it no longer becomes his choice to seek help. You could then contact someone who will assist you in intervening with this colleague. This could be a family member, a trusted close friend and colleague, or the department Chair. The intervention should occur in a prearranged time and location, at a time when the colleague is not intoxicated. Be prepared with documentation of their problem behaviours, an explanation of why you think they need help, clear expectations for accessing help and consequences if these expectations are not met, and have an assessment pre-arranged. Again, the PHP can assist with advice on intervention and assessment.

It is not easy for us to approach colleagues in difficulty. We do not want to intrude, or embarrass a colleague. We worry that we may be wrong in our concerns. We assume that they may already know how to get help, if needed. We worry about possible anger or negative repercussions. We worry about ruining their reputations or their careers. In fact, done in a compassionate and caring manner, it may be the best thing we ever do for them.

Domestic Abuse in Medicine

I had previously written an article on identifying and treating abused women in our medical practices. A female colleague wrote to me about the emotionally abusive relationship she is currently in, demonstrating great courage and strength in writing and sharing a situation usually undisclosed. She told of how her husband constantly criticizes her and her family, blames her for anything that goes wrong, and puts her down in front of the children. Domestic abuse is hidden, the best-kept secret in families. Domestic abuse is everywhere.

Here are some of the disturbing facts:

- Domestic abuse is present in 25-50% of all relationships. Emotional and verbal abuse are much more common.

- 50% of assaults result in injury, but only 4% of these injuries are diagnosed correctly as a result of abuse.

- The incidence of abuse is higher in pregnancy, marital separation, or if child abuse coexists.

- 25% of women who attempt suicide are abused.

There are six types of abuse:

- *Psychological* – the victim is frightened, harassed, and verbally threatened.

- *Emotional* – victim is criticized, belittled, and blamed.

- *Economic* – the victim is made financially dependent.

- *Sexual* – the victim is forced into coercive, non-consenting sexual contact.

- *Physical* – the victim is physically hurt.

Legal – the victim is engaged in vicious legal and court battles.

Women physicians are not immune. Women physicians also find themselves in unhealthy relationships, such as ones in which they are criticized and diminished; isolated from family and friends; dealing with alcoholics in denial; physically beaten; living with a partner who she supports because he is chronically unemployed, in debt, and expects to be bailed out. As I saw more of these situations in my practice, my question changed from "Does it happen?" to "Why do they stay?"

Four years ago, I conducted a survey of women physicians seen in my office in a randomly chosen week. I saw 19 women that week, all of whom agreed to complete the survey. The unpublished results showed that 37% of the women had experienced some form of abuse in their relationship:

- 50% of them described the abuse as Emotional.

- 10% as Physical.

- 10% as Sexual.

- 10 % as Mixed.

The frequency of the abuse was described as:

- Daily by 30%.

- Weekly by 20%.

- Monthly by 40%.

- A one-time-episode by 10%.

Only 50% of these doctors had spoken to a physician (me) about it; 20% had shared it with a friend; and 16% had told a family member.

Abuse is all about *power* and *control*. It often starts out as a non-violent form of control. When the power imbalance is established, it can escalate to physical violence, often gradually. The Cycle of Abuse has three phases:

Phase 1: Tension Building. This is the "calm before the storm," in which the early warning signs are there, the conflict is building up, and abused person feels like she must walk on eggshells.

Phase 2: The Explosion. The abuser "loses it," erupts and explodes, and acts on his rage.

Phase 3: Honeymoon Period. The abuser reverts to acting calm, is back in control, and behaves in a sweet and charming manner.

One of my female physician patients, a surgeon, likened these phases to the stages of an abscess formation. First, something gets under your skin and is irritating. You try to wall it off and contain it, but it overwhelms your system and continues to accumulate and enlarge. It ruptures and drains, but if the source is not eliminated, the abscess slowly recurs.

Women who are victims of abuse are not wimps. Women physicians who are in abusive relationships are extremely successful, highly motivated, financially independent, experts in their fields, and appear together on the outside.

Why do bright, independent women stay in such a situation? It is not because they are weak, or because they like it. In my survey:

- 47% hoped it would get better.

- 26% stayed because of the children.

- 11% were concerned about being able to cope financially on their own.

- 6% feared violence from their partner.

- 6% worried that no one would believe them.

- 4% worried that their partner would not cope well without them, and are caregivers.

It is not just women physicians who can be in such situations. In the past six months, I have seen three male colleagues who are also in abusive relationships. All of what I have stated above applies to them too.

If you are in such a situation, remember that:

You have rights; the right to; be treated with respect, be heard, say no, come and go as needed, have a support system, have friends and be sociable, have privacy and a space of your own, and have a separate identity.

- This is not your fault. You did not cause this.

- You can't change them; you must change yourself.

- Educate yourself about your legal rights and responsibilities.

- Prepare and pack. Make and gather copies of all important documents: bank statements, income tax statements, investment statements, marriage and birth certificates, passports, and wills.

- Remove yourself from the cause of harm, if you feel in danger.

- Find a safe place, with family, friends, church, crises lines, and shelters.

- People will listen, and believe you.

- Develop support systems. Avoid isolation.

- Stay healthy. Eat, sleep, exercise. Care for yourself.

- Seek therapy. Improve your self-esteem, and learn to be appropriately assertive.

- Regain your sense of humor and play.

As a profession, we need to educate ourselves, and not assume that these things do not happen in our midst. Domestic violence thrives on ignorance.

So Sue Me: Dealing with the Stress of Litigation

At a recent medical meeting, I ran into a classmate from medical school. She told me how she had just received a letter from the College of Physicians and Surgeons of Ontario, regarding a patient complaint. The patient was threatening to sue her as well. She was not sleeping well, felt nauseated all day, and was tied up in fear and guilt. She wondered how she was ever going to cope with this.

The threat of litigation hangs overhead for all physicians. There is nothing like a lawsuit or a complaint to tap into our self-doubts. It is said that every physician will experience this at some point in his/her career.

In 1996, a Canadian Medical Protective Association (CMPA) survey revealed that 95% of physicians experience stress during the complaints process. The most significant stress occurs upon initial notification of the complaint. Physicians experience a range of emotional, physical, and behavioural symptoms. About 50% reported that these interfered with their personal and professional lives. However, after resolution, only 25% felt that the stress was completely eliminated. The results of this process are long lasting. One of my patients described it like a trauma, with resultant Post-Traumatic Stress Disorder.

Emotional symptoms include anxiety, lack of trust in patients, frustration, anger, disbelief and sadness, loss of image, loss of power, helplessness, and a sense of loss of control. Physical symptoms can be insomnia, exhaustion, headaches, palpitations, gastrointestinal symptoms, or generalized aches and pains. Behavioural symptoms include sleeping problems, use of alcohol or medication, a need to talk about the complaint, internalization, social withdrawal, a need to get away from the office, a decrease in working hour, a wish to leave the practice or profession, and family disruptions.

SECTION TWO

Before there is even a complaint, it is good to put a preventive program in place:

- Understand the Process. Identify issues that may lead to complaints; know and follow the rules that govern the practice of medicine; understand the complaints process.

- Preventive Strategies. These focus on good patient care; foster clear, timely and effective communication; appropriate and complete documentation of medical records; early recognition of dissatisfied patients; maintenance of knowledge and professional behaviour.

- General Coping Strategies. Develop and maintain effective stress management techniques; learn to care for yourself, and develop a supportive personal and professional network.

During the complaints process:

- Stay in control. Identify and focus on what you can control.

- Contact and notify the CMPA. This will be your most valuable resource for information and advice.

- Imagine you are studying for your qualifying exams. This is just another similar challenge. Study the case, pore over the file, take notes, learn the details. Know your stuff. Be prepared. Look and act confident.

- Do not avoid the problem. Force yourself to review the records and chart. Read letters from lawyers, the College, and the CMPA. If you know a problem may arise, write down details of the situation as soon as possible after it has occurred.

- Do not avoid the lawyers. Take calls from the lawyers, and return them promptly. Meet with your lawyer. Do not worry about being embarrassed or being judged by them. This is their job, and they can help you. (It is like a patient with Erectile Dysfunction—embarrassing for them, not for you.)

- Set priorities. Let go of other things, to allow yourself to focus on this.

- Be prepared for the hearing. Ask yourself questions, and prepare answers. Learn about the process, layout of courtroom, order of events, where to sit, how to address the judge, and how to testify. Know where you are going, and be on time. Dress in business clothes. Be calm, clear, and credible.

- Understand and identify roles. Your role is to explain and defend yourself. Their role is to question you. Do not personalize this; they are just doing their job. (Note: This is a different role than in patient care.)

- Use the "Best Friend" technique. Imagine it is your best friend who is being grilled. Stand up for yourself, as you would for them.

- Accept your feelings. Express anger productively. Push yourself past your fears. Balance your doubts. Identify and limit self-recrimination. Do not allow yourself to sink into despair.

- Take a break. Set limits for the time you will devote to this preparation. Take time off from this process, and remind yourself of what is going well for you.

- Talk to trusted colleagues. Reach out to colleagues who know, like, and respect you. Recognize they still feel the same about you. Focus on your feelings, not details of the case. Ask for support, not for advice.

- Stay connected. Do not isolate yourself from friends, family, or colleagues.

- Learn and use relaxation techniques.

- Understand and expect the spiral nature of this process. It waxes and wanes, and will not improve in a linear manner. It is like a marathon, not a sprint. Pace yourself accordingly.

- Continue with work as before. Know that there is no reason to doubt your self. None of your patients or colleagues doubt you; there is no visible mark or stigma of the lawsuit.

- Take care of yourself. This will allow you to be able to do your best through this process.

We Are Care Givers, not Care Receivers: Barriers to Help

I received an email from a colleague I had never met. He recognized that he was experiencing burnout and probably had depression. He needed help but had not yet gone to see a psychiatrist. "I know that I should do something about this, but cannot bring myself to do this. Something holds me back."

Many physicians find it hard to be a patient. Being both a physician and a patient is a unique therapeutic situation. In the usual medical model, the physician is the healthy, wise, trained person in the room. The patient is the sick one, and is naive and untrained in medicine. In the circumstance where the patient is also a physician, both sides of this model are changed.

I am amazed at how ill my colleagues can be, and still continue to practice well. The work arena is often the last to be impacted. Most doctors put off coming for help. No one comes to see me because they have a couple of free hours in their week; and have nothing better to do! Most people come when they hit a crisis. They become so depressed they cannot get up in the morning. They get a letter informing them they are being sued. A patient dies on the operating table. They come home, and their family has moved out.

How can we wait so long, in such distress? It is because we are intelligent, and as such, use high level, intellectual defences, to protect us against having to deal with difficult emotions. These defences include:

Denial; "I'm all right, there's no problem."

Minimization; "OK, maybe I am not at my best, but some of my colleagues are actually doing even worse than me."

Rationalization; "It's just because I have not had a holiday in the past year."

We use reaction formation, a defence in which we form a reaction, and give to others all the care and attention we would like to receive. One of the most serious defences is sublimation, and working harder. When things are difficult, it can be easier to stay at work and keep busy, so we do not have to stop and think. Work is a good defence, because it works well. We get away with it because we can always find more work to do, we like our work and can do a bit more, and because this is socially acceptable. People do not worry about us; in fact, they often think we are better doctors because we work more. Defences are important to identify, because they are the main reason why doctors do not come from help when we first require it.

There are many other reasons colleagues cite as why they hesitate to come for help. There is a stigma of mental illness, even more so in medicine than in the rest of society. As physicians, we are supposed to be strong and capable. Being ill is felt to be weak, a failure. We feel a sense of shame and guilt, as if we should have tried harder to feel better. Our personal insecurities come to the surface, and we fear judgment and exposure. We are not sure about the prognosis of a diagnosis of mental illness.

There are the practical problems, too. We think that we cannot take time away from our practice, or from our patients. We worry that our patients will not get the care they need, or that our colleagues will have to work even harder to make up for our absence. There is the fear of lack of confidentiality, especially if the psychiatrist you will be seeing is in a hospital setting. Sometimes, we do not even know where to go to for help. In addition, we have real concerns about the impact on our ability to obtain life and disability insurance afterwards.

Seeing another physician as a patient can bring about a struggle for control. As physicians, we like to be in control. Handing over this control to someone else is not easy, even if we choose whom this someone else will be. I discuss this with all patients when I first meet them. I tell them about my own experience as a patient when I was very ill with a twin pregnancy, having developed the HELLP Syndrome, an uncommon obstetrical complication with hemolysis, elevated liver enzymes, and low platelet counts. I recall some colleagues, who were in charge of my care, asking me what I thought they should do as my condition worsened.

I did not want to make this decision. I could not, as I was too ill, and I felt that this was too big a burden to take on. I want to reassure my patients that, while they are informed colleagues and I want to hear their opinions and preferences, they are given permission to be patients in my office and can leave the responsibility of the decisions to me.

It is very hard to accept help. We are care givers, not care receivers! This is a new role for us. Feeling as you do is not the norm. Don't settle for this; you deserve to feel better again. Reach out, and make the first step. Call for an appointment. There is no failure in getting help. In fact, the failure is in not getting help when we need it.

It Must Be Nice

It is September, and the air is cooler, and the leaves are just starting to turn orange and red and yellow. Everywhere there are signs of increased activity as people come back from holidays and return to work, and children get ready to head back to school. I can't help but think about those who are not returning to anything for a change—the colleagues who are not well, and are required to take time off. This is an amazingly difficult time for them. Their experiences are rarely addressed, and I thank them for sharing their remarkably similar stories and allowing me to write about them.

Previous chapters have addressed the common personality traits of doctors and how it is so hard for us to acknowledge that we are not doing well, and need help. It is hard to recognize signs and symptoms of stress, burnout, depression, anxiety, and addictions in ourselves. It is even harder to reach out, beyond the stigma, the fears and insecurities, the guilt and the self-reproach, to get help. For some, getting treatment requires a minor adjustment of their schedule to include regular appointments, therapy, and possibly medication. For others, it requires a much greater adjustment of schedule, as they are too unwell to continue to work and are advised to take time off. This is never a light decision-either by me as the treating physician, or by the physician-patient who has huge responsibilities in an already under-resourced field.

By the time colleagues comes for help, they have often waited longer than the average patient. As a result, they are often much more ill, with severe symptoms. Finally admitting their difficulties is a huge step, and there is a great sense of relief at not having to pretend any longer, or to have to continue to act as if all was fine.

However, despite this relief, it is rare that colleagues accept the advice to go off work easily. There is the initial guilt of having gotten to this point, for having "allowed" it to develop, and being weak and having failed in some way. Then, there is the guilt of having to leave their patients and practice "in the lurch" at the last minute. As well, there is the guilt of adding to the burdens and responsibilities of their colleagues, who they know are already working at their maximum capacity, but will likely be required to pitch in even more during their absence.

There is also fear—fear of not being believed, especially since there is no visible or tangible disability such as a heart attack, a diagnosis of cancer, a broken limb, or a back injury. Other fears include the fear of being judged by colleagues as being weak and not cutting it as a doctor, limiting their career as a result. There is the fear of not being believed and being thought to be of faking it in some way; of being penalized; of being ostracized. There are additional fears of lack of confidentiality, concern about impact on their license, and concerns about not being able to get disability insurance.

Yet, even after acknowledging that they are very ill, and not functioning at their best, limited in decision making abilities, and doubting themselves at work; and then finally agreeing to taking time off, most doctors do not just go home. In fact, it is quite the opposite—they reach deep within for the "final push" and squeeze out the last remaining ounce of energy to clear off their workload as much as possible, plough through their booked appointments, complete their paperwork, clear their desk, and do as much as they can before they leave. This productivity is understandable in view of their large sense of responsibility, but makes their going off work even harder to understand for their peers.

The first week off is often spent in a state of shell-shock. They are usually amazed because, in sharp contrast to their last week of work, all they can manage is to eat, nap, and sleep. Then, the real work begins. There is time for reflection of what happened, and of what needs to be modified. There is the realization that they do not know how to relax and will need to learn. Self nurturing is not a skill that comes as second nature. There is the need to switch from taking care of others to taking care of them-selves. This, again, can lead to guilt, as the physician feels that

"I should look depressed while out in the community, to justify my absence." It feels wrong and dishonest to have some fun or to do something enjoyable. Yet, this is exactly what one needs to re(learn). Nowhere is it written that the treatment of depression is to lie in bed all day with the covers pulled up over one's head.

One of the most painful aspects of this journey is dealing with the varied reaction of their colleagues. There are those who are kind and caring and supportive—it is not easy for us to accept this care. Of course, more difficult are the less caring responses. Some colleagues say nothing, do not contact us, and effectively ignore us. While this silence may be a (often unconscious) sign of their discomfort in speaking of this topic, it is perceived as uncaring and dismissive, or a clue to their anger. In one hospital department, a doctor was hospitalized with a heart attack. His colleagues came to visit him daily, and sent cards and notes and flowers. Another colleague in the same department was hospitalized on the psychiatric unit with severe depression. Not one of his departmental peers sent a note or a gift or came to visit!

Some responses are more overtly lacking in understanding or empathy. After a doctor was advised to go off work, she returned to her office for the rest of the week to tell her colleagues and to complete as much as she could before she left. As she was finally leaving the hospital on Friday afternoon, a colleague casually called out to her "Good bye. Have a good time off…it must be nice!" Others tell me of similar comments, supposedly in jest, about "being lucky" to be able to take such a "long vacations," especially if the timing of the illness coincides with summer or Christmas. Some doctors have been told that this is their fault— that they deserved this, that they created it, that it was avoidable and self-imposed, or even that it was the result of greed. Other direct comments refer to surprise at their being ill when they had been so productive in recent days prior to the leave, suggesting they did not believe them and felt they were faking, not recognizing this as the "final push" I described earlier. While some of these reactions are experienced prior to the leave, they also occur when the doctor returns to work. It is helpful to anticipate them, and plan a response, so one can deal with it without feeling hurt, defensive, or judged. Interestingly, many doctors tell me that, while this is painful to experience as a recipient, they admit that their own attitudes in the past were often similarly judgmental. Insight is often only attainable when one is touched by this personally.

This highlights the need to continue education within the medical profession to nurture the development of a compassionate understanding, which allows open discussion, early recognition of illness, and supportive collegiality. The process of educating ourselves, and our colleagues, is bumpy and painful...but it has begun.

CULTIVATING PEAK PERFORMANCE

David vs. Goliath: Dealing with Insurance Companies

I recently received a letter from a colleague in Ontario, expressing her frustration with difficulties encountered regarding her disability insurance coverage. Having been part of her provincial medical association insurance program for over 20 years, she had applied for increased insurance as her income has increased and she felt she required greater coverage. This was denied to her, since she had undergone a period of disability of three months a few years back during a time of personal crisis which was now resolved. The insurance company was still willing to insure her, just not increase this coverage. She felt this decision by the insurance company was confusing and unjustified. She felt she was being discouraged from seeking help, even penalized for acting responsibly to ensure her health. She appropriately stated in her letter that physicians needed advocacy in this area.

From my experience in working with colleagues as patients, I am acutely aware that this is a real problem. Colleagues repeatedly tell me stories of how, after seeing me, a psychiatrist, they are unable to obtain disability insurance coverage, or that their premiums are inflated, or that their disability coverage does not extend to any disability due to any psychiatric illness.

Many physicians similarly feel penalized for getting help. The concern about the potential impact on their ability to obtain disability insurance is cited as one of the main reasons that physicians do not come for help when it is required. This is a problem, since it actually delays treatment, and can create a worsening of the condition, leading to disability, a lengthier resolution, and time off work. In fact, in the majority of cases, I can unequivocally state that the person's likelihood of requiring time off work is markedly decreased when they seek and receive psychiatric help in a timely fashion, and gain insight and learn strategies to cope with their situation.

There have been several attempts to address this issue for physicians in recent years. The Canadian Psychiatric Association launched a committee to understand this issue and identify ways

31

to better manage it, and has created a Task Force on Disability Insurance Issues, in response to concerns by members about practices by the insurance industry related to access to coverage, claims processing procedures and reporting requirements by psychiatrists. The CPA Section on Physician Health will work together with this Task Force to further these efforts. The CMA Centre on Physician Health and Wellbeing has identified the need to advocate for Canadian physicians and support their insurance needs as one of its priorities.

During my year as President of the Ontario Psychiatric Association, I decided to explore this issue further on behalf of my colleagues. I realized that each provincial medical association has negotiated a separate policy for their members, and there is little consistency. However, there is work being done to push for increasingly more comprehensive and affordable coverage. It has evolved in the past 50 years, to offer coverage from medical school to retirement. Medical professionals at an early stage in their training and career can now obtain full insurance protection at a low cost, without having to qualify medically and undergo the health history, or blood or urine testing. This is great for current medical students and residents. However, this does not address the specific issues of currently practicing physicians, who obtained insurance before this opportunity was available. These colleagues have experienced great difficulty in obtaining such coverage.

Some colleagues state problems in obtaining coverage after having sought help from a psychiatrist. In fact, some psychiatric residents who undergo therapy as part of their training are also denied coverage, without any evidence of a psychiatric diagnosis. This was justified for patients with burnout, anxiety, or depression, since these diagnoses represent a large proportion of the reasons for claims. It was also likened to chronic back pain—if someone has a history of back pain, the insurance company also excludes them from further disability claims. Yet, it is not entirely similar. While a few physicians have serious illnesses leading to permanent disability, this is not often the case. Most colleagues usually learn much from the therapy, and gain insight and skills to manage their illness better so they do not become disabled in the future. There is some evidence to show that highly educated patients recover quicker and more fully than the average population. We need to have this demonstrated clearly and credibly to the insurance companies.

It appears that there is little documented evidence of the problems that colleagues tell me they have encountered when dealing with insurance companies. There is some question by some organizations that these incidents even occur.

The efforts being taken by those working in the area of Physician Health to advocate for the insurance needs of physicians are just the beginning of a long path. It is an onerous task, a bit like David taking on Goliath. The insurance companies are very large and powerful. However, there is strength in numbers. This is of at least two types. Firstly, numbers and data. (If you have had an experience with an insurance company that supports the suggestion that there are inherent problems, please let me know. Give me a short, clear summary, so I can build a case. I will not be able to present your case individually; but rather create the data that is currently lacking that can lead to further action.) Secondly, the numbers of people advocating on behalf of physicians needs to increase, so "David's" strength increases. We can help the momentum slowly build towards better mutual understanding.

Time Off Is an Investment

I am looking ahead to the holidays. For the first time in years, I have decided to take two whole weeks off. The kids are not back to school until later in January, and so I guiltily decided to stay home with them. I know this is my choice, but I feel badly about this. I feel that I am letting my patients down, too.

They say that misery loves company, and feeling guilty is a form of (self-induced) misery! I know that I am in good company. Many doctors are considering a similar break if they can, but feel uneasy about actually doing so.

Much of this reaction comes from our personality traits. We are very dedicated and perfectionistic professionals. We conscientiously attend to the needs of our patients, and have difficulty delegating this. We are highly responsible, and feel very guilty if we do not meet these responsibilities. Add to this our sense of self-doubts, and we find ourselves unable to justify a decision based solely on our needs. In fact, we have learned, perhaps perfected, the art of deferring our own gratification. No wonder I feel guilty! I am doing something that goes against my basic personality.

Another factor is the culture of medicine. This reinforces that the right thing is to always do what is best for the patient. It encourages deferring our own needs, values self-sacrifice, and a selfless focus on our work. This culture underlines that it is weak for doctors to take time for themselves or admit that they may need this. It reinforces that a doctor who keeps longer hours is a better, more committed, and more dedicated one.

In addition to our psychological traits and the culture within medicine are the expectations of our patients. Patients have learned to expect prompt and immediate care. For years, doctors have delivered this; but in the changing and limited health care system, it is becoming harder to do so. A recent angry letter to a newspaper came from the friend of a patient who had his hip surgery delayed "because the surgery conflicted with the doctor's latest vacation plans." It was inaccurately implied that the doctor took endless vacations, and constantly changed his operating schedule, and it was stated that "this type of treatment and lack of concern...is disgusting and inhumane and borders on the criminal side of malpractice." We all reel from and work to avoid this type of feedback.

The reality is that we need to take holidays. Just as we are told during the airplane safety demonstration to put on our own oxygen mask before we assist anyone else, we need to ensure that we take care of ourselves so we can continue to be available for our patients. We are of little use to them if we are barely coping, at the end of our threshold. Holidays must be seen as an "investment," a small bit of time and energy devoted to our own needs, so we can meet the needs of others. In reality, most doctors take few holidays. In my practice, the self-employed physicians take an average of two weeks off a year. Colleagues who are on salary or have benefits rarely take the full amount of holidays to which they are entitled. Let's start by encouraging each other to take vacations, and offer to cover for each other.

Go ahead and book your holidays. Do it responsibly with regards to your practice, so you can manage the guilt and not let it hold you back:

Recognise that you need a holiday, and that this is an investment.

Plan your holidays in advance. Use the Tarzan Rule. Just as Tarzan swings through the jungle, not letting go of one vine without having another in hand, do not end a holiday without having booked the next one.

Once planned, block off this time. Do not book patients, appointments, or procedures during this period. Patients cope better with being given a later appointment, than having an appointment cancelled.

Arrange to have a colleague cover for you while you are away. This works best as a reciprocal arrangement. If you do not have such a colleague available, look for a locum, or hire an agency to offer coverage in your absence.

Tell your patients you will be away, and give them appropriate notice. Do not be defensive, apologetic, or give unnecessary explanations. Sound confident, and state that things will be fine while you are not there. This gets easier with time. You may have to "fake it 'til you make it" at first.

Let your patients know who will be covering while you are away, and how to best reach them.

Anticipate reactions from patients. Most of them will be happy for you and understanding. Expect some to be angry. Acknowledge their anger, allow them to express it safely, and just restate your plans and that you know it will be fine.

Recognize that you are a role model for your patients. You are modelling healthy behaviour, by setting limits, setting your health as a priority, and ensuring time for self-care.

Deal with the guilt. Guilt is what we feel when we do not feel we are meeting our own expectations. Since we set these expectations, we can reset them. Acknowledge this feeling, and identify it as guilt. Recognize there is no need for it, and consciously work to let it go. Remember the *Rule of Thumb* about Guilt: If you are thinking of doing something that makes you feel guilty, that is the very thing you should do! If it were unreasonable, immoral, unacceptable, unethical, illegal, it would have been censored out already. If it remains a viable thought, it is because it is reasonable and does not call for guilt.

Once you are finished work on your last day, start having fun immediately. You are now on holiday already. Get into this mind-set, and maximize your time off. Put a smile on your face. Plan to enjoy this time, with your family, and friends.

Return to work happy and rejuvenated!

The Tarzan Rule

For many years, I was privileged to be a member of the faculty for Psychiatric Update for Family Physicians, speaking on the topic of physician health. This was a series of highly acclaimed land-based and cruise conferences for family doctors, the brain-child and creation of two psychiatrists, Drs. Tony Sehon and Alan Buchanan, of Vancouver, BC. It was that rare and successful combination of fun and education, and quickly became an annual event for many repeat attendees.

I had a conversation with Alan during a quiet moment after one of the courses, discussing tangible tips to help reduce our stress in medicine. He told me about the Tarzan Rule, a simple yet brilliant concept based on how Tarzan swings through the jungle, never letting go of one vine until he has another one in hand. The rule is all about making sure we have similar vines, which are future holidays or at least, specific time booked off work, which allows us to swing (manage effectively at work) between holidays. Essentially, the more vines one has, the lower the stress experienced.

It started as an idea they heard from one of their course attendees, on a Caribbean cruise. He described to the conference group how he had completely changed his approach to organizing his holidays, now always having the next one planned. This new way was dramatically different than what almost every family physician in the course was doing—waiting until they felt completely burned out and only *then* booking a holiday.

Alan and Tony immediately built upon this idea. They made up a visual Tarzan picture to show in their Physician Stress talks in future conferences, and were actively encouraging the docs in further courses to start thinking about planning their holidays using the Tarzan rule. The concept really caught on, and doctors were coming up to Alan and Tony in later conferences, telling them this concept was one of the most valuable things they had learned in the entire conference (usually 15-18 hours of material). There were always lots of positive stories telling how the concept had worked for them. The spouses also highly praised this concept, and felt it made a positive difference in their family life. Medical colleagues would strive to be healthy "Tarzanians," a concept solidly associated with the *Psychiatric Update* conferences.

In fact, the early adopters of the Tarzan rule began to use the *Psychiatric Update* courses each year as a "vine," going to different places in Canada each year and cruising in different areas of the world. This helped them establish a routine of always having another vine or two planned before they let go of the present (vine) holiday. Often, they were motivated to start definite scheduling with their offices for the next conference even while on the current cruise, recognizing that planting a vine in the future was a good idea since the education at these conferences was top level, definitely practical, and highly entertaining.

Alan and Tony generously allowed me to use the concept in my presentations, not just with their conferences, but in all my talks. Our mutual goal is to share the Tarzan Rule with as many colleagues as possible and assist them in their efforts to remain healthy.

I love the Tarzan Rule, and encourage colleagues to use it not just for holidays, but everything they do that makes them feel good, healthy, and strong. Plant the next vine!

- Don't end a holiday without having another one booked.

- Don't end a run without knowing when you are going for another run.

- Don't end an evening with good friends without knowing when you will be seeing them again.

- Don't end a visit to the spa without booking your next visit there.

- Don't end date night without knowing when you can go out again without the kids.

- Don't end the golf game without booking the next tee off time.
- Don't take the last slope of the day without knowing when you are taking the family skiing again.
- Don't uncurl yourself from that chair and stop reading without knowing when you are coming back for the next chapter.

Continue this list on your own and personalize it. Identify the things you do that make you feel reenergized, and make a commitment to having one more booked before you end that one. Follow the Tarzan Rule, plant as many vines as you can...and stay well.

SECTION THREE

OPTIMIZE TRAINING TO PRODUCE RESULTS: BEING A DOCTOR

.

SECTION THREE

Asserting Yourself

Assertiveness is a trait that enhances our success in all aspects of our life. Yet, for many physicians, being assertive does not come easily or naturally. Most of us have been taught to be "good"—to work hard, listen well, try to please others, be pleasant and easy going and considerate, and not focus on our own needs because that would be "selfish." This is essentially right, and such behaviour has helped get us to where we are now. Such hard work and focus on others has contributed to our studying hard, getting good marks, getting into and through our training in medicine, and becoming well-regarded physicians.

While behaving like this is not wrong, restricting our behaviour to this is not entirely right. This has helped us get this far, but we need to learn more skills to achieve further success. Being assertive is one such skill.

A colleague in the department told me about her difficulties in her private practice with her partner. While she is responsible for half of all of their expenses, she does not feel that she has half of the rights within the office. Her colleague makes most of the decisions. The office staff do things her colleague's way even if she asks them otherwise.

Asking does not come easily to us. We often feel that we should not have to ask, that others should just know what we want and/or deserve and give it to us. I don't think that there is anything much harder than asking for what we want. At the start, you need to define what it is that you want to say. It helps to be clear, direct, and succinct. Watch out for preambles and modifiers, words and phrases that make it easier and softer, such as "If that's alright...I hope you don't mind if...sort of...I may be wrong about this but..." since they dilute or discount the point you want to make. Plan out your thoughts, and keep it short and simple and quick. "I would like my charts filed in this manner." This will be your bottom line.

You have to make yourself heard. I am sure that you can recall coming with a great idea in a meeting, only to have someone else bring it up a few minutes later and get the accolades. Why is this? Bring up your point in a simple declarative statement, instead of a question. "I suggest that ..." instead of "Do you think it would work if we..." Also, you don't have to wait until everyone else has spoken. Interrupting someone can work to your advantage. Take as much time as you need, and speak confidently. Don't let others interrupt you; ignore the interruption if it occurs and just keep on talking.

Use the *Mirroring* and *Broken Record* techniques to state your point assertively. Listen to the other person, and then respond with a two-part statement. The first part is the "Yes, I hear you," in which you mirror by restating what they have just said or what feelings they have just expressed, so they know you have heard them. You reflect back their point of view without necessarily adopting them. Yet, don't stop here. Continue on to the second part of the statement, in which you stand your ground and state your bottom line. Thus, whatever the other person says, you can agree with something of what they have said; and then state your bottom line. You can repeat this over and over, as they bring up new points, like a broken record. This has at least two benefits— your point is reinforced as you say it repeatedly, and you do not go off on a tangent since you keep coming back to your bottom line and make your point.

Once you ask for what you want, it is helpful if you can reframe it, to show the other person how it can also benefit them. Often, the needs of both parties are not mutually exclusive. Highlighting how it helps both of you can help you work together towards the same goal, instead of remaining at odds.

Just asking for something, no matter how clear and direct, is not always enough. There are two more factors that help meet the goal. Set a deadline, by which your stated expectation must be met. "When do you think you can get this done by...I would like to have this completed by..." Then, define a consequence if this deadline is not met. A consequence can be a serious, but often it is not dire, just a way to ensure that you can follow up. "If I do not hear back from you by tomorrow afternoon, I will call you."

Sometimes, you just need to decline or disagree. It is okay to say no. Follow these three easy steps:

1. Open your mouth.

2. Say "No."

3. Close your mouth.

We often continue on to explain, apologize, and make excuses in an attempt to please and retain approval, yet this is not always necessary. "No." is a complete sentence.

To summarize, here are some concrete steps in asserting your needs:

• Recognize when you need to ask for what you need.

• Do your homework and find out what is reasonable, possible, and works best.

• Ask or decline clearly and directly.

• Show how what you want will also help the other person meet their needs.

• Set a deadline, by which your expectation must be met.

• Define a consequence if the deadline is not met.

• Then, stop talking.

The key is to be strong and assert your needs, without being destructive. State your needs calmly and surely, to ensure that you will be heard. Speak confidently, and if you don't really feel confident at first, "fake it until you make it."

It gets easier with practice, especially when you see the results it brings!

The Four Letter Technique: Managing Anger & Resolving Conflict

There are times when we are appropriately assertive, but others do not seem to listen to what we are saying. We all may know someone like this, who just becomes angrier, louder, and appears very threatening. When there is a problem, he or she blames others for it and calls them incompetent and stupid. Sometimes, this may make us angry, too, but it is usually easier to just pull away and let things be.

However, while avoiding this overtly angry reaction is easier at the time, it is not easier in the long run. If there is something you need to say, it is not easier later. There are two parts to this situation: dealing with your anger, and then dealing with your colleague's anger.

Let's start with dealing with your own anger. Sometimes, we think we should not be angry. We are more comfortable with being patient, tender, and compassionate. Anger, as a feeling, is always appropriate; it is how you express it that makes it more or less acceptable.

The best way to start to address your own feelings is to acknowledge and identify what it is. Some of us are so uncomfortable with "negative" feelings, such as anger, that we deny them and so do not even know when we are angry. Understand your own anger. Anger is always a secondary response; it can follow feeling hurt, afraid, sad, disappointed, and embarrassed.

Then, we need to learn ways to express this. Try creating an anger vocabulary. Take a piece of paper and write the word "ANGER" on top, in big, bold letters. Then, underneath, write all the ways you can think of to express your anger, and other words and phrases that connote the same feeling. Listen to what others whom you like and respect say when they are angry and add this to your list. Ask family and friends you feel safe with what they would say when angry. Be open to looking for other suggestions in movies and books. You cannot express your feelings if you do not know how. (If you have time, while you are at it create a vocabulary for other feelings, too. Instead of "Anger," make several columns, with the words "Mad, Sad, Glad, and Afraid" on top, with grateful apologies to Dr. Seuss, and find more ways to express those feelings.)

The *Four Letter* technique is a great tool. Using these words and phrases, write out your angry feelings in a letter, addressed to the person directly. Say exactly what you want to; do not hold back or edit your thoughts and feelings. This is not a letter that you will ever send. This is crucial and bears repeating—do not *ever* send this letter. If you have done this properly and really said what you felt, this is never productive for anyone else to read. While it may sound like it captures your points perfectly at the time, it is too intense for anyone else to understand. Rip it up. Press delete. When you start to feel the same again, write out a second letter, then a third and then a fourth. By the time you get to the fourth draft, you are calmer, your writing makes more sense, you have probably found a more balanced perspective, and you can decide *if* you need to address it further.

Venting your feelings to a highly trusted family member, friend, or colleague may help, too. If, after this, you feel you want to address the issue productively to the person, use "I" and "Me" statements to express how you are feeling. Decide what point you want to make. If there are many, limit yourself to one point at a time.

What if the other person is angry? How do you deal with that? First of all, anticipate the process. Then, whatever their response is, you will be better able to deal with it, and not be caught off guard. The best way to defuse anger is to agree. You do not have to agree with all that they are saying, but you can always find some aspect of it to agree with. Sometimes, all we can agree with is that they are angry; this is enough. This can help to calm things down.

If they continue to express anger, yell, or hurl names, you can call them on their behaviour. "I beg your pardon...That sounds like an insult. Did you mean it that way?"

Remember, you do not deserve to be yelled at. Ask them to stop. Say "Please stop yelling. I will discuss this later in private." Or "Stop. I do not like to be yelled at."

Continue on to set limits. Here are some steps:

- Acknowledge the situation. "It's clear that you are upset."

- Commit to your involvement. "I am happy to work with you to address it."

- Describe what behaviour you do not like. "Words like…When I hear you say…"

- Describe the effect of this. "I get defensive...I shut down...I don't want to work with you."

- Give your preferred scenario. "I would prefer it if you could calm down and tell me what you would like…"

- Mutually positive consequence. "That way, we can work together to sort this out…"

There are different levels of setting limits. Start with a polite request. This often works. You may have to progress to increased verbal intensity, and match their voice tone and pitch. Finally, you may have to state a consequence "I will report this behaviour to…" Be sure to follow through.

Overall, we have control in this situation, if we choose to use it. You have no control of their behaviour. However, you can control how you react to it. Also, you can control how much it impacts on you. If you woke up that day planning to have a good day, do not hand over control of how your day goes to, of all people in your life, this person. Have the day you want to have.

SECTION THREE

Pull a Logan: Learning How to Say No

While it is true that adults teach children, it is also true that adults have a lot to learn from children. Teaching is not a one-way process. Children have a special, innocent way of viewing the world. They have taught me to laugh more, enjoy the moment, be curious, use my imagination, accept differences, and be spontaneous. More recently, I learned that they have skills that we sometimes have to re-learn as adults.

I had just finished a workshop for colleagues on communication skills, including assertiveness, which is the expression of feelings and needs, asking for what you want, and stating views with directness and honesty while being respectful of others. We had discussed how being assertive can help to strengthen relationships, and prevent stress arising from conflicts and resentments. We explored why it is so hard to set limits or say 'No.' It can be difficult for us to be assertive, to stop pleasing others and start to set limits clearly to protect our time for self care. We feel we have to justify our decisions, to ensure people do not judge us as uncaring or lazy. We do not want to be disliked, or be seen as bossy or rude. We do not want to risk upsetting others. Sometimes, we feel that our own needs are not as important as those of others. Some of us are very uncomfortable with conflict, and will acquiesce just to avoid conflict-laden situations.

In the workshop, we described strategies to become more assertive in a productive way. "Three Easy Steps to Saying No" (see *Asserting Yourself*, p.42) were demonstrated to an appreciative audience!

After the workshop, I visited my sister and her family. I watched my young nephew, Logan. At two years of age, he is the picture of confidence, strutting about his space, knowing exactly what he wants, without compromise. He could be the poster boy for assertiveness, being persistent, determined, and clear about his viewpoints. In fact, at times, he can save energy and state his wants clearly, without even speaking. He has this amazing gesture of raising his bent right arm from the shoulder and pushing his elbow out, shrugging off an unwanted suggestion. When asked what that meant, Logan unabashedly explained "I don't want to!" Time to leave the park and go home? Out goes the elbow. How about peas with the mashed potatoes? There goes the elbow again. Can Aunty give him a kiss? Not unless she gets past the elbow!

Recently, I have started sharing my nephew's technique of limit setting with patients—calm, clear, direct, and honest. Without excessive emotion, it clearly communicates what he is or is not willing to do.

I ran into a colleague last week, who proudly told me how he had "pulled a Logan" with success. After recognizing that he was feeling overwhelmed, he had finally reorganized his responsibilities to lessen the burden, and was starting to enjoy exercising regularly, have time for friends and family, and explore a new hobby. He was asked to assume a more senior position in the department. Keeping Logan in mind, he did the "elbow elevation" and was thrilled with the results. "I just looked him in the eye, and confidently and calmly said 'Absolutely not!'" Look for opportunities to use it; it works!

SECTION THREE

Brag: Promoting Yourself Effectively

I see colleagues in the hospital moving ahead, being promoted, and being recognized for their achievements. I am happy for them. Yet, I also see others who work hard and achieve a lot, but seem to be passed over; as if no one seems to know anything about what they have achieved. One colleague confessed that she feels like she is still a resident, working hard in the trenches, while others get the glory. How can she improve this situation, and have her achievements recognized?

The quick answer—promote herself! Brag is not a four-letter word.

Many physicians work hard to please others, yet retain a sense of insecurity and self-doubt. They feel uncomfortable with approval or positive feedback. We assume that if we work hard, we will be recognized and rewarded. We learn to remain quiet about our work and achievements, and downplay our successes. We even let others take credit for our achievements. We feel the right way is to "Just do a good job; let others notice us." Such attitude and behaviour is seriously limiting your career, as you may be finding out.

A colleague recently applied for promotion in his academic department, and jokingly stated that one needed to have a narcissistic personality to properly fill out the forms, which required you to say how great you are and how recognized your work is. At a workshop on preparing a promotion application, another colleague remarked how this application process felt so awful and demeaning, that; "Managers should find out what we do and how well we do it, and just give us the promotion when they realize we deserve it."

The message is the same—one must learn to promote oneself. This is important in all parts of daily life at work, not just when we are formally applying for promotion. In her book, *Brag! The art of tooting your own horn without blowing it*, Peggy Klaus speaks of the myth of modesty being a virtue, and discusses how it holds one back in the workplace, in building relationships, and in feeling confident and powerful. She gives some specific suggestions to communicate your talents and accomplishments, without sounding like a walking billboard.

Tell colorful stories about yourself. At a meeting or function, never be tongue-tied again. Have a "brag bag" ready—a list of interesting information about things you have done, fascinating trips, unusual hobbies, challenging or funny situations you have been in. Relay these stories with passion and use specific details.

Talk to people, not at them. Ask others about themselves, really listen to their answers, and make good eye contact. Look for cues to bring up your own experiences when the timing is right, and sow productive seeds of information about yourself, and what you are doing.

Show excitement about your life. This is enjoyable and contagious. Cultivate this feeling, with words like "I am so happy about..." Use humor to your advantage.

Use the "best friend" technique. Imagine you are your best friend. Consider how you would introduce yourself to everyone, with positive support. Plan to meet at least three new people at each meeting or event you attend. Smile at others, and establish and maintain eye contact.

Get involved, serve on committees, help out, and meet key people in the organization. Once you meet these important people, follow up on the contact. Send a quick email, a post card, or a thank you note. I once met the Chair of the Psychiatry Department at a very prestigious university at a conference where I presented. He made a few complimentary comments at the end of my keynote presentations, until someone more important than me came and whisked him away. When I returned home, I sent him a quick postcard thanking him for his kind words, and made sure to write my contact information. He replied with a request for me to present Grand Rounds at his university!

Write your own impressive bio. Include things you are very proud of. Make it crisp and punchy. It is amazing how often others will use it word for word. Sum up your work or reputation in one word or phrase; this makes it easier to connect you to that achievement.

Tell others when you achieve something, your peers, and those in authority. Do not be shy about telling about an award, a paper you wrote, an idea you had, or a challenging patient you helped. Accept praise and compliments, without downplaying or dismissing them. Say "Thank you."

Self-promotion is undeniably a necessary skill in today's medical workplace. Everyone is working hard at their own job, doing more with less in today's health care environment. If you don't tell others what you are doing, they may be too busy to find out.

Doctors & Money

It's tax time—that time of year that we all look forward to... putting behind us, that is. I can feel the associated sense of stress myself, and it is definitely palpable in the office among my patient colleagues. There are those who have not filed a return for many years. Some colleagues have filed a return but not paid outstanding taxes for the past few years. Others did not pay their quarterlies and will be scrambling this year. Some of us made more than we expected in the past year, and now have to pay more taxes than expected, unsure where this money will come from. Even those of us who paid our quarterlies on time, have things in order to file the return, and do not owe any extra tax, still find this process very stressful.

Doctors have an interesting relationship with money. We want it and need it, but don't feel comfortable talking about it. In the culture of medicine, doctors are supposed to work because we feel a calling, and are dedicated and conscientious. The money is to be seen as secondary, and we are discouraged from any discussion on this matter. In our social culture, doctors are seen as rich and privileged, and so are not widely supported in any conversations about financial remuneration.

Our thoughts and feelings about money are also a product of our past experiences. Take a moment to reflect what money meant to you and your family as a child, because it definitely impacts how you feel about money now. Was money an issue for your family? Did your family struggle financially? Were you limited because of financial reasons? Can you think of an incident as a child in which money was a factor? Recognize that this incident will color how you experience money now. For example, there was a period in my life when money was tight. My father died unexpectedly in a car accident when I was eleven years old. There was no will, and it took some time to clear up the finances. I am sure that this is why I now still keep small stashes of money around "just in case," even though it is no longer an issue. I have $20 bills tucked away in my office drawer, in my car glove compartment, in my kitchen drawer, in my home office desk, in my bedside table…you get the point. (Now that my teenagers have found most of my spots, it is safe to write about them!)

Why do we get ourselves in debt? It is not always easy to understand how such a group of intelligent, highly educated, high earners manage money so poorly. Sometimes, it is due to reasons of our control——change of jobs, illnesses, accidents, or changes in relationships. However, for some doctors, it is unconsciously self-inflicted. We are too nice, want to please others, and seek approval——this makes it hard for us to set limits, we can't say no to people we care about who want to buy something extravagant, and it makes us behave generously with others (e.g., picking up the whole check at a restaurant). We may feel insecure and need to prove ourselves–this may lead to a need to buy things that make us seem more secure and successful, such as expensive clothes, jewellery, cars, and homes. We are good at delaying gratification, and put things off throughout our training——as a result, we can feel entitled to getting exactly what we want and feel we deserve once we finish, and overextend financially. We compare ourselves to our friends who chose other professions and started working years earlier, and want what they have achieved. This continues during our working life, as our work is very stressful and takes so much from us; we can justify "treating ourselves" afterwards. Being self employed does not help at times, as we can always justify an expense by telling ourselves we can work harder to pay for it later.

This is compounded by the current reality that many medical students graduate with a significant amount of debt. One of the students in my mentor group, who came to medical school after another graduate degree, recently graduated with over $200,000 in debt! Tuition costs have risen and continue to do so. Bursaries, scholarships, and grants have not kept up with this increase. Financial institutions are happy to offer credit cards, loans, and lines of credits to these young future earners. It is now the norm for medical students to spend much of their studies living on credit.

This situation is a true source of concern. Money is one of the main reasons why doctors experience such a high degree of stress. They make personal purchasing decisions that put them in a critical financial situation. Thinking about this causes significant stress. They have to keep working and earning to maintain this lifestyle. As a result, they cannot make the changes they may need to make to decrease their stress, such as book a Monday morning off from clinical work when they return from a holiday to catch up on paperwork, phone calls, lab results, mail, and emails. In fact, many feel the need to take on extra patients, shifts, and call to keep up with their expenses. This extra workload and stress can lead to fatigue, irritability, medical errors, burnout, and depression.

The lack of knowledge about finances, or a high debt load, can be a source of shame and embarrassment for some of us. Ironically, it prevents us from reaching out for the financial help or advice we need. Sometimes, we may not even know the basics of money management—setting goals, knowing how much we are earning or spending, budgeting, having a savings plan, paying off non-deductible debts first, and investing wisely. If you feel this way, it may help to know that you are in good company. However, remember that even though you do not know much about money, you have everything it takes to learn!

It is said that the best time to start managing your money was yesterday. The second best time is today. There are many good resources for financial advice available to physicians either through your medical associations, your accounting services or your banking institutions; call them. Luckily, April always ends, and May brings with it the hope and promise of a new year with more financial control and serenity.

They Who Laugh, Last: The Value of Humor

"Incontinence Hot Line…can you hold please?" The boys laugh out loud again. As they get dressed to head out into the cold morning of an Ottawa winter, they glance at the board in the mudroom. I have a dry-erase message board there, and every night after my sons are in bed, I write a new joke there. It has become a ritual after all these years; I look for short snappy jokes every night, and the boys look for them every morning. A fabulously fun start to our day.

"Laughter is the best medicine." This is something we all know intuitively. We know that we enjoy being with people who make us laugh, that a good laugh is rejuvenating, and that it makes us feel better. Scientific research backs this up. Dr. Lee Berk of Loma Linda School of Public Health in California has found that laugher lowers levels of stress hormones such as cortisol and epinephrine, and strengthens the immune system. Dr. William Fry from Stanford University showed that twenty seconds of guffawing gives the heart the same workout as three minutes of hard rowing. Laughter lowers blood pressure, oxygenates your blood, and increases your energy level. A study at the Oakhurst Health Research Institute in California of heart attack victims followed over a year showed that of a group who watched comedy videos for a half hour a day, 10% had a second heart attack, whereas 30% of those who did not watch the videos had another heart attack. Dr. Michael Miller from University of Maryland Medical Center found that blood vessels expanded while watching funny movies and contracted during serious movies, reaffirming that laughter benefits blood flow to musculature and reduces blood pressure.

It has been said that the average child laughs about 500 times a day. By the time we get to adulthood, it drops to about 5-15 times a day. Many of us do not even get this daily dose. Yet, laughter is simple, easy to do, and cheap. It is one of the best stress reducers around, and is worth seeking in a proactive manner.

OPTIMIZE TRAINING TO PRODUCE RESULTS

There is a misguided assumption that humor at work is just playing, or goofing off, and is immature or unprofessional. In fact, we are starting to recognize that the opposite is true; that making work fun leads to sustained peak performance, productivity, collegiality, and professionalism.

There are still myths to dispel:

- Being humorous means we don't take our jobs seriously. In fact, it just means we don't take ourselves too seriously, and allows the focus to shift from the job to the people doing the job.

- Being humorous undermines our authority. In fact, it can strengthen your sense of confidence, control, and authority, and allow one to lead successfully in a stressful situation.

- Being humorous is not for everyone. Some people just aren't funny and should not try. In fact, one can learn and develop this skill with interest and practice.

- Being humorous means that you are immature. In fact, there is intelligent, witty humor.

- Being humorous prevents people from being successful. In fact, successful people understand the value of humor, and have the confidence to use it productively.

- Being humorous is unprofessional. In fact, humor can be, and should be, expressed with great sensitivity and respect.

Laughter in the medical workplace can be an amazingly positive tool to make work fun, reduce job stress, create a sense of team, energize colleagues, and improve physician morale. Here are some ways to look for humor and to add it consciously and productively within a medical setting:

- Create a humor bulletin board for the office or clinic. Encourage everyone to contribute. You may need to assign someone to monitor it to ensure appropriate humor. Look for cartoons, jokes, or quips.

- Put old cartoons from the board every month in a scrapbook or album for continuing enjoyment.

- Subscribe to a humor site or software service that provides a joke a day.

- Subscribe to humor magazines such as *Stitches*, or *Punch*.

- Put humor anthologies in the waiting room for patients to enjoy.

- Have a fun dress-up day in the office that is still professional and appropriate—e.g., Ugly Tie Day, Ugly Shoes Day, Pink Shirt Day.

- Have your own version of a Cartoon Caption contest in the office/clinic. Send around a cartoon, invite captions, and vote on the funniest.

- Use humor to promote upcoming events like meetings, birthdays, and holidays.

- Look out for good jokes and share them with colleagues.

- Be sensitive to when any kind of humor is not fun or appropriate.

"They who laugh...*last*."

No More Excuses: Exercising to Stay Healthy

Yesterday afternoon, I finished my workout, had a quick shower, and headed out to meet a colleague over coffee. Interestingly, he arrived a few minutes later, looking refreshed and calm. He apologized for the short delay, explaining that he had just started to work out again and felt great, and really wanted to keep it up. He hoped that I did not mind that he had tried to fit in the exercise before our meeting. Of course not; in fact, I was truly impressed. "100% of the physicians at this table exercise regularly!"

We spoke of the clear benefits of exercise and how we know all about this, but admitted that we did not always find time for it over the years. He had just joined a gym at the hospital, and found it was easily accessible and convenient to drop by on the way home. I agreed that if time could be saved, that made it more likely for us as physicians to do this regularly. I confessed guiltily to my current exercise routine—I have a personal trainer come to my office just after my last patient has left, 2-3 times a week. At the start, she set me up with an exercise mat, exercise ball, a graduated set of free weights, weight bar, and rubber bands, and now mercilessly puts me through my paces. This saves me the transit time, and so allows me to fit in this workout when I just have 45 minutes, instead of requiring two hours. I run every morning on my own for the aerobic part of the workout, and actually stick to it because I am accountable to her.

This got me thinking more about doctors and their exercise habits. I wonder what the actual percentage of colleagues who exercise regularly really is. Doctors know all about the benefits of exercise—preventing heart disease, high blood pressure, diabetes, osteoporosis, cancer, depression, and obesity. Exercise is not only associated with positive physical health, but better mental health, too. The psychological benefits of exercise are genuine. It is associated with a general sense of fitness, improved self-esteem and confidence, and a positive outgoing attitude Athletes speak about the psychological "high" and the adrenaline rush. Recent studies have documented that exercise increases serotonin levels, just like the SSRIs, thereby leading to some elevation of mood. As well, exercise has been shown to increase the number of neurons in the hippocampus, another possible factor in the alleviation of a depressed mood. As doctors, most of us know that the recommended amount is 30-60 minutes of exercise 3-5 times a week. Yet, we do not always practice what we preach, to take care of our own health needs.

Bortz, in 1992, described the health behaviour of physicians from a specific US clinic and found the exercise habits to be typically better than those of the general population. Erica Frank and her colleagues (*JAMWA*. 2003; 58: 178-184) reported on the exercise habits of US women physicians, and found that nearly all (96%) reported getting some exercise; the median time spent being 3 hours per week; the main activity being walking, followed by gardening, biking, swimming, running and aerobics. Half of these women exercised enough to meet the above recommended amounts.

However, this high level of activity is actually not borne out by my observations of colleagues, both within my practice and within my medical community. Some experts explain the healthy results from the research cited above by postulating biases in the studies—that physicians who were proud of their activity level were more likely to respond; that the ones who were not so healthy did not have time or energy to respond to the survey; or that physicians responded by stating what they would like to be doing (and will be starting tomorrow!), not necessarily what they were actually doing.

Understanding barriers to regular exercise for physicians involves an understanding of our basic personality traits. Physicians are very dedicated and conscientious, and so have other things to do that seem higher on the list of priorities. Exercise is seen as "something just for ourselves, a luxury to be enjoyed when we have earned it." Our sense of responsibility makes us feel guilty when we feel we are not meeting it; thus we feel guilty to be exercising when there could be other things we could do with that time. We are people-pleasers; thus we will try to do things that other want of us first. We have had such good practice in delaying our gratification; it is easy to slip into this again in this regard. Our perfectionism can set us up to fail. We start an exercise program and want to do it perfectly, each day. Then, when reality intrudes and we miss a day or two, we feel we have failed and can abandon it entirely. This is an interesting aspect, as we often see that the colleagues who do regularly maintain fitness, do so at an exceptionally high level, such as running marathons. Our self-doubts and insecurities are key factors that can prevent us from exercising. Starting an exercise program when we are out of shape feels impossible; it is easier to do things we know we are good at (such as work). It is embarrassing to be seen in exercise gear in the middle of a busy gym, and have those amazingly fit people there watching us struggle as we figure out how the machines work (guaranteed to tap into those insecurities!). It can be hard to justify the time and money involved, as we are not sure we are deserving of this.

There are other barriers, more real ones that result from the lifestyle of medicine. Research by Verhoef et al, 1992, cites marriage, especially with children, as the main barrier to exercise for women physicians. Johnson et al, 1990, described other barriers to include work pressures, perceived lack of time, and lack of personal discipline.

Here are some general tips for starting and maintaining an exercise program:

- Recognize this is not a luxury, rather it is an investment. Taking time for yourself makes you more available to meet the needs of everyone who is counting on you.

- See it as something you want to do, not a chore or duty. Regularly remind yourself why you want to exercise. (I have yet to achieve that runner's high; I exercise so I can eat.)

- Make it a part of your day, just like having dinner. Thus, it is not *if* you have time to exercise, but *when* you will do it.

- Set aside the time; book it in to your schedule like you would a patient.

- Start slowly, and set a series of achievable goals, so you can feel progress and success.

- Don't wait to get motivated. Push yourself to start when you said you would. Once the action happens, the motivation will kick in.

- Try the Five-Minute Rule—promise yourself that you only have to do it for five minutes and then you can stop if you wish. Chances are that you won't want to stop after five minutes, but it helps to know you could.

- Allow a degree of flexibility. If you cannot do the full routine that day, just do what you can. If you miss some days, just start again as soon as you can.

- You don't have to do this perfectly. Just because you could do it at a high level, does not mean you need to, or should do so.

- Don't get discouraged. Some changes occur immediately; others take more time to be evident.

- You have nothing to prove to anyone else.

- Enjoy the workout; choose something fun.

- Choose something you like to do, and that you are physically able to start.

- Exercise with a partner who is not judgmental can help to make it fun, and keep you sticking to it.

- Take the time to exercise without guilt. If you are in a relationship, express appreciation, and offer the same to your partner.

No one method or routine works forever. Vary the workouts regularly, or enjoy it for as long as you can. When it no longer works, look for something else that will work, for this new phase of your life.

Remember, you are worth it.

OPTIMIZE TRAINING TO PRODUCE RESULTS

I invited colleagues to share what they do to maintain exercise in their life. Here are some actual suggestions that colleagues have offered:

- Join a health club that is accessible—at the hospital, close to work, or on your way home.

- Hire a personal trainer. Mine comes to my office, but they can come to your home, or work with you at the health club.

- Use exercise as a form of transportation. Bike or run to and from work.

- Choose the stairs over the elevator as often as you can.

- Park your car as far away from the door as you can.

- Go to bed early and wake up early to exercise before the rest of the family is awake.

- Watch television as you work out; the time seems to fly.

- Watch a good movie while you work out. That way, you will want to exercise the next day to see the ending.

- Don't come home until you have completed your exercise. Stop by the club on the way home; it seems harder to take time for exercise once you are home.

- Hire a sitter daily to free up a couple of hours to work-out, if your kids are young.

- Join a gym that has child care.

- Put the treadmill in the play room so you can supervise and work out.

- Exercise with the children—swim, go for hikes, bike rides, chase them at the park.

- Go for a walk or run, while you are waiting for your children to finish the music lesson or hockey practice.

- Join an activity with your partner, such as dance lessons.

- Learn yoga or Pilates. Look for opportunities to practice this during the day.

- Sign up for lessons for a sport or activity—tennis or skiing lessons.

- Join an active club, such as a running, biking, or cross-country skiing group, so the group can help to keep you motivated.

- Reward yourself with new gear from time to time.

- Dress like an athlete. Fake it until you make it!

If all else fails, try *The Every Excuse In the Book Book: How to Benefit from Exercising, by Overcoming Your Excuses*, Bean Fit, 2005. Jeannie "Bean" Murdoch offers fun yet rational responses for 120 of the more common excuses people use for not exercising. The hardest thing to rationalize may be paying $24.50 to knock down a carefully cultivated arsenal of excuses!

Addressing this now allows you to beat the rush for New Year's resolutions, or even better, to choose something else to resolve then!

I Thought You Wanted to: Setting Boundaries to Manage Your Time

It's October, and we are all busy and back to work after the more relaxing summer. There is so much to do, getting the children back to school or university, the start of the academic year and lectures to prepare, committee meetings being scheduled again, and clinics and offices full of patients. There are more emails to read and respond to, and I am finding myself at the computer late in the evenings, just to get all the emails dealt with and off my desk. Yet, I realized that no sooner would I sent them, than the replies would start to arrive. I was obviously not the only one working longer at my computer! We were all trying to get our work finished, but it seemed as if technology was conspiring against us to keep the work ongoing.

I thought back to my undergraduate university days in the early 80's. One of my friends from high school was actually working towards a degree in Leisure Studies, as it was assumed that computers and increased technology would free us all up so much, and we would likely need someone properly trained to assist us in deciding how to use our new-found leisure time. Little did we know that it would actually eat into our leisure time, blur boundaries between home and work, and add a sense of time pressure to all of our work. Gone are the days when we would take time to write a letter, drop it in the mail, have it received a few days later, allow a few more days for reflection and reply composition, and then have it mailed back to us. Sending someone a letter meant that we could expect a reply in two to three weeks. The reply now seems to be expected within two to three hours! Computer emails take enough of our time; add to that the BlackBerry's ability to bring them to us immediately, as well as other things like podcasts, FaceBook, Twitter, Skype; and it seems amazing that we actually have time for anything else. At times, I miss the face-to-face interactions, the sound of someone's voice at the other end of a telephone, the smell of an envelope in the mail.

As the emails start to fly back and forth this fall, I am noticing a curious thing. Colleagues, friends, and family are responding to a line I have added to my email signature that reads "There is no need to respond to this email during the evenings or on weekends." Now, before you start thinking how brilliant this is, I have to tell you that I did not entirely think this up on my own. A senior colleague and mentor had once added a line at the end of his email to me on a Friday afternoon, reminding me that I did not have to reply immediately. I felt an immediate sense of relief, and asked him for permission to add a similar line at the end of all of my correspondence. I have been impressed to see that many people notice this line and often experience a sense of relief similar to my own when I first read it.

Many have added comments on that line at the end of their emails:

- I like your statement, "no need to respond to this e-mail..." Great for quality of life and balance.

- I love the signature file; great reminder not to go overboard with all this technology.

- I LOVE the little sentence at the end of your message...yeah that's the right attitude...

- What a great idea that last line is, thank you.

- P.S. I really like the note at the bottom about not replying evenings or weekends! What a great idea!

A friend who runs her own successful small business wrote "This is something we should ALL encourage—as a small business owner, it's a huge challenge not to be online 24/7, but IMAGINE...if we all worked towards that (your line)...wow, we might have our lives back!"

One of my favorite responses was "Although I'm going against the last line in your signature...I want to comment right now, as I won't have a chance tomorrow! Great idea, and I am going to start adding it to my emails, too."

We are all conscientious, dedicated, and hard-working. We want to do our best, meet our commitments, be seen as reliable and gain approval—yet sometimes, this means doing so at our own expense. Our training in medicine has reinforced such behaviour. This sometimes makes it difficult to set limits and boundaries, and decide that we have done enough for one day and that "Good enough is good enough." It is not easy to stop, knowing there is still more we could do and more to be done. Yet, the reality of our lives is that there is always more to be done, with expectations to do it faster than ever before. We have to start assessing our achievements by our own realistic expectations, not the idealistic ones of others.

I had a big "Aha" moment one day when I was setting up a wellness program in our university, spending long hours, wanting to do it perfectly knowing it had never been done before. I was telling a senior colleague how it was a lot of work on top of my usual work and I was not sure how much longer I could keep working at that pace. He told me something I will always remember; that he was impressed by how much I had achieved in five months, creating what he had expected would take five years to do. Then he said, "But I thought you *wanted* to do this." Simple words, but life-altering for me. I realize that when I do something, even if it means making sacrifices or stretching myself, others don't think more about it and simply assume that I must want to, that if I did not want to, I should say something or stop. It is up to me to decide how much to work and when I choose to do it in my day.

Yet, how do we start to set realistic expectations of ourselves when we have never done so before? I use the *Best Friend* technique. I ask myself what I would sincerely expect of a friend/colleague that I truly like, respect, and admire, and then do the same for myself.

SECTION THREE

I am pleased if the simple message at the end of my email gives others a chance to pause and reflect. It makes me hopeful that perhaps we will someday learn how to rein in this technology, use it to make things better, but not allow it to take over life. In the meantime, I continue to work hard to set and maintain limits, learn how to set automatic evening/weekend/vacation responses, and turn off my BlackBerry and the computer during evenings and weekends. It's amazing how much more time I have—for people in my life, for fun, for me!

Get Organized: How to Control Clutter & Regain Order

I recently hosted an evening meeting of the Ottawa branch of the Federation of Medical Women at my home. Despite the frigid winter temperature, there was a great turnout as we all welcomed the opportunity to enjoy each other's warm company.

The guest speaker was a professional organizer—a perfect start to the New Year! She spoke about how many professionals feel life is busier than ever, that it seems that there are never enough hours in a day, and that time is wasted looking for items. We can all benefit from taking back control and reducing the clutter in our lives, so we can focus on what really matters. It is not about appearing neat and tidy; rather the goal is to be able to function well within that environment.

It is interesting to consider why we let things become cluttered and disorganized. We thought back to a time when we actually felt in control—surprisingly, for many of us, it was during our first year away from home at university! This is when we had only a few possessions to manage, had a limited space to manage them within, and lived alone so we could manage it ourselves. Thus, it follows that we become increasingly disorganized as we gain more things, have more space to put them in, and have other people who live there and use and move things around. The extra work and responsibilities we have gained over the years do not easily offer us the time and opportunity to become organized. As well, we are responsible people; we could not possibly get rid of something we may use/need it in the future…so it accumulates. Growing up with parents who were immigrants or lived through the Depression makes it even harder to "throw out something that is still perfectly usable." For many doctors, being a perfectionist, having OCD, or ADD can add to chronic disorganization. It is helpful to understand why being organized is not easy to achieve, and nice to know that we are not alone.

The SPACE methodology is a good tool to becoming organized, and can be applied in any room or situation.

- *Sort*: The initial goal is to sort and group like items together in broad categories, so you can first see just what and how much you have.

- *Purge*: Decide whether to toss it, give it away, sell it, put elsewhere, or keep it. (The clutter test helps in this decision. Ask "Do I love it, use it, or gain energy when I see it?" If not, it is clutter and can be removed. A great tip is to keep a photo as a reminder of items we keep for purely sentimental reasons.)

- *Assign a home*: Decide exactly where the item will be placed, and ensure the location is accessible and safe and easy to return to.

- *Containerize*: Once you know what you are keeping, put it in a container to limit it, and allow easy retrieval and cleanup.

- *Equalize*: Maintain with regular evaluation and periodic tune-ups.

These are ten tips to organization, from OrganizeMe101.com:

- Think before you buy. Do I need the item? Do I love it? Where will I store it? Is it worth storing and maintaining?

- Store things close to where you will use them.

- Store things conveniently. If it is too much work to put away, it won't get put away.

- Use these four sorting boxes as you tidy; Put Away, Give Away, Sell, Throw Away.

- Do a "clutter patrol" of your living areas nightly, and put things back in place.

- Eliminate regularly; don't let clutter build up.

- Try putting away a few decorative accessories; you may still like the look.

- Find people or agencies to donate to, and use them often.

- Have a "maybe someday" bin; put things here first if you can't throw them out, and date it. If you haven't used something in six months, maybe you can live without it.

- Limit the number of horizontal surfaces in a room; they are magnets for clutter.

None of us manage this perfectly, but it can be easier than it feels at times. Similar to weight loss; if you don't want fall victim to "yo-yo" organizing, you will need an internal attitude adjustment and ongoing de-clutter maintenance. Yet, the reward and calmness that comes with achieving a better level of organization and feeling more in control is worth the effort.

SECTION THREE

With a Little Help from my Friends: How Friendships Nurture Us

I drove home this evening with a smile on my face, singing along with the radio, thinking of how lucky I am. I had just spent a wonderful evening with a dear friend—a deluxe manicure, a relaxed meal on the patio of a restaurant on a perfect summer evening, lots of laughs, and quiet shared thoughts and support. I have known her for over twenty years; and there have been times when I saw her daily, and times when years went by with no contact. Yet, I always knew she was there, available, understanding. We have seen each other through the rigors of medical training and subsequent professional decisions, as well as the joys and crises of our personal lives—marriage, pregnancy, babies, adolescents, separation, divorce and remarriage, and now planning children's weddings! No matter how long it has been since we last met, we always pick up where we left off, and the intervening time becomes irrelevant.

I reflected on other friends and the light they have also brought to my life over the years. The friend who planted my annuals for me one year when I was away a lot in the early summer. The friend who left a lemon meringue pie on my doorstop when I was recovering from an illness. The friend who signed us both up for a yoga class. The friend who is blunt and tells me when I need to lose weight. The friend who mentors me and connects me to others who can help me in my work. The friend who sends me orchids randomly for no reason. The friend who patiently taught me to mountain bike. The friend who makes me laugh until I cry.

Life in medicine is exciting and fulfilling, but full of demands and requires us to be responsible much of the time. We are busy, tired, and easily drained. Friends feed our soul. They are the difference between a lonely and a lively life. Friends can be a lifeline at times of transition, such as a change of job, end of a relationship, when the children leave home, or when we are ill and needing chemotherapy. They are there to support, nurture, and listen.

There is a lot of research to support the benefits of friendships. Friends protect our bodies. It is known that people with friends recover quicker from illness, use fewer medications, and need to see their doctors less often. A University of Chicago study showed that socially connected people have more robust hearts. Researchers from Carnegie Mellon University showed that the more social one is, the less susceptible one is to getting the common cold. Teresa Seeman from Yale University followed the death rate of 10,000 seniors over five years, and found that more social ties correlated with a lower likelihood of death.

Friends also protect our sanity. A landmark study led by Laura Klein of UCLA showed that women respond to stress by "tending and befriending." Under stress, a cascade of chemicals, including oxytocin and estrogen, is released, which leads women to bond. This in turn increases oxytocin levels, which lessens stress and leads to calming. This helps to understand why many women in medicine naturally turn to other female colleagues, and form groups of female colleagues to cope better with work-related stressors.

There are no rules or limitations about who can be a friend. They can be from childhood or from a current phase of life. They can be male or female, the same or opposite gender from you. They can be of a similar age, or a different generation. Cultures or traits can be similar or entirely different. One can be drawn to the other from the start, or dislike each other at first. Friends can live close together or several thousand miles apart.

Our personality traits as physicians help us be a good friend. We are responsible and conscientious, so will follow through on promises and intentions reliably. We are people-pleasing, so do caring, thoughtful, and lovely things for others. We can delay our own gratification and put our friend's needs first. However our traits can also limit us as a friend. We can be seen as controlling. We feel guilty, and can do things for others out of guilt and resentment, especially if we have put off our own needs. We have self-doubts and do not believe others really like us or can feel easily threatened with a sense of failure if our friends succeed.

While our personality traits can limit our ability to be a friend, other factors interfere too. Our work can keep us too busy to have the time to cultivate and maintain friendships. We juggle other priorities and responsibilities, such as time for spouses, children, parents, and communities.

What makes a good friend? Relationship experts, Drs. Les and Leslie Parrott, describe ten traits for enduring friendships.

A Good Friend:

Makes time; In times of crises, and in the middle of the mundane.

Keeps a secret; Trust is essential, they are "human vaults" who make you feel safe.

Cares deeply; Care allows a friend to enter your world and feel your pain.

Provides space; Offers room to breathe, to be individual, is not oppressive

Speaks the truth; Is able to, honestly yet respectfully, tell and hear the truth, despite the pain. This is your conscience, the first one you turn to in a moral dilemma, who asks the questions you want to ignore, so you do not stay in denial and helps to force reality.

Forgives faults; Knows you and likes you anyway! Can overlook and forgive minor faults.

Remains faithful; Is loyal and does not desert you in bad times when you fall.

Laughs easily; Can share a laugh, finds the same things funny, is fun, and great to be with.

Celebrates your success; Is not jealous, resentful, competitive, or threatened. They lend a hand to help, and to applaud. This is your best promoter, great before interviews, or when plagued by self-doubts.

Connects strongly; Feel common interests and share similar phases.

We need to work on being a good friend, before looking for a good friend. Dale Carnegie advises that you can make more friends in two months by becoming interested in other people, than you can in two years by trying to get people interested in your self.

The summer is a great time to nurture friendships. Patients are away on holidays, so clinics and offices may be less hectic. Department and office meetings slow down. There is less teaching to be done. Colleagues are on holidays, so rounds are often cancelled. The days are longer, so bright evenings offer promise and possibilities. This provides more time to be available, and to work on your friendships.

Think of a close friend who means a lot to you. Show her you care by reaching out and contacting her. Book regular activities together, such as golf games, bike rides, lunch, or a day at a spa. If she does not live close by, plan to meet in the near future, and stay connected via regular phone calls or emails. Once you initiate contact, use the Tarzan Rule to keep it going—do not end that contact without booking one more. Anticipate and allow for change over time, and do not take it personally. Be open to sharing feelings and trusting her with your hopes and fears. Talk openly, and acknowledge problems, apologize and forgive. Listen carefully, and be thoughtful and empathetic. Expect to have fun together. Plan to laugh until you cry, let loose, know that you are safe with her. Thank your friends for being there—call, write, or just say thank you. Remember, to have a friend is to be a friend.

SECTION THREE

Recalculating: Stop & Explore Options

I sat down to work on this chapter, eager to get started, write out a few points and take time to flesh it out. The computer turned on, froze, and then went blank. For a few seconds, my mind froze and went blank, too. Now what? My initial thought was to worry, as this was the evening that I had put aside to complete this chapter, and all the other evenings were already booked full of other plans.

Then I recalled something I learned during a family road trip we recently enjoyed. On one occasion when we were using the GPS to direct us as we drove into a new city, we noticed the gas tank was almost empty. We were on course, following the directions, and heading to our destination, but then pulled into a gas station to fill up. The GPS stopped and, with its sexy male voice in that fabulous British accent (Nigel, we call him), stated "Recalculating." It then took stock of where we were now, where we needed to go, and revised the route…all with no emotion. The GPS did the same again, later when we had to make a detour for construction—no fireworks, anger, or recrimination from Nigel; he just stopped for a second, assessed the problem, and offered a new option. Brilliant, simple, efficient, and effective.

Our family uses this simple tool every chance we get. When something does not work out, we now just say "Recalculate" and it reminds us to stop and calmly look for another option.

This makes complete sense. The number one cause of stress, regardless of the situation, is feeling a lack of control or choice. Thus, the number one solution is to challenge this perception, identify what we do and do not control, and focus on what we can control. It is a fact of life that things will not go as planned—that's the part we do not control. The part that we do control is that we do not need to become overly emotional, remember that there are options, and look for them. In cognitive therapy terms, we are reframing the situation, looking at it differently, and are thus better able to cope in it and remain in control.

OPTIMIZE TRAINING TO PRODUCE RESULTS

September is a busy month in every household, full of new beginnings, hope and promise. The kids are heading back to school and university. That means back-to-school shopping for school supplies, new lunchboxes and healthy snacks, and fall clothes that fit. The academic year starts up in the Faculty of Medicine, with its hectic teaching schedules, meetings and conferences. There are hockey tryouts, band auditions, and exercise classes to register for. New seasons of theatre/opera/ symphony/ dance subscriptions are starting. Of course, things will not happen as planned. There will be schedule conflicts, too many drives to manage in an evening, things forgotten until the last minute, and missing and misplaced items. Each one of these situations can be an opportunity to recalculate!

This evening, with my computer not cooperating, I decided that I would try to do the same myself. I just "recalculated" and reassessed my options. As my computer sat there frozen, I could hear Nigel's voice encourage me "Recalculating." I remembered the old days, before computers, rummaged through a dusty drawer for a pen and some paper, and started to write down the points by hand. However, my thoughts were gone. What was I going to write about? Again, as I started to worry, I remembered to recalculate and decided to focus on that and share this simple tool with you! This chapter flowed. Brilliant, simple, efficient, effective. And all with little energy lost to unproductive emotion!

The Platinum Rule: Giving People what They Need

A colleague in my office was recently shaking her head as she spoke about her children's reaction to Halloween and all the candy they had collected. She recalled her own experiences as a child—she came from a family with modest means, where all the basic needs were covered but there was little money left over for extras. That meant there were no treats on a regular basis, no dessert, no special clothes, no outings to the movie theatre in town. She would wait with enormous anticipation for Halloween when there would be an unusual surplus of treats in the house. Every year, she would be disappointed when her mother would limit them to two treats when they returned from trick-or-treating, and then put the rest away to be rationed out over the following months. When her children returned from being out for Halloween this year, she told them they could eat as much candy as they wanted. She could not believe it when they each enjoyed only two or three small treats and then wandered off, replete. She had just given them what she would have loved to have had herself—unlimited access to candy—and was stunned at their lack of appreciation of the offer and lack of interest in taking her up on it. Yet, as we discussed it further, she realized that her children had regular access to such treats and so did not see her offer as special.

I told her about my "Platinum Rule" that I had created over the years (platinum being more valuable than gold). This Platinum Rule supersedes the Golden Rule that we all learned as children—Do unto others as you would have done unto you. All of the great world religions teach such a message, and this forms the basis of our current concepts of human rights and equality. It is an essential moral principle, requiring knowledge, respect, understanding, and imagination to place ourselves in the other person's situation and visualizing how to act in a way that we would like to have someone act with us.

Yet, the Golden Rule is not always the best possible mode of action. It is ideal to take it one step further—not just consider what we may need, but to also consider if the recipient needs that same thing, as well as what else the recipient may need more. It accommodates their interests and desires, not ours.

While the Golden Rule states "Treat others as you want to be treated," the Platinum Rule suggests "Treat others as they want to be treated."

I saw this occur in my own family and parenting. I am one of five sisters, and would have loved more of my busy mother's time and attention. When I had my own three sons, I resolved to give them just that. One evening when the twins were three, and their older brother was four years old and had just started school, I decided that I would give them each a nice long bedtime cuddle, for twenty minutes each. One of the twins loved every minute of it, wanted his head and back rubbed and protested when our time was up, bargaining to have just one more back rub. The other twin enjoyed our time together, seemed happy to get some hugs and chat about the day, and wished me a good night as I got up to leave. I went in to my older one's room, who gave me a hug, and after a couple of minutes asked "Can you please leave now, Mom? I'd like to go to sleep." I quickly realized that it was my need to give them each twenty minutes; that was not in fact what they each wanted or needed. Luckily, they were all able to tell me their differing needs, and I was able to hear them.

The Platinum Rule is a rule worth keeping in mind during the holiday season. As I think about gifts to give to friends and family, I try to think about who they are, what they mean to me, and what they may want or need. (The only exception is still giving my sisters things I want…so I can borrow them back some time! I quote the Golden Rule for that.) In our busy lives, the people we love and care about do not always need more stuff and things. They work hard and earn well; they have most of what they need. They would also appreciate our time, care, help, thoughtfulness, and our full attention. Over the holidays, I encourage you to reach out to family and friends; connect with them; turn off your laptops and smart phones; and make time to just be with them, enjoy time together, and have nothing else you have to do. The resultant rewards of rich connection will be a mutually treasured gift, and allow us to return to work recharged.

Checking Your Gas Gauge; How Full Is Your Tank?

It's back to work after the holidays. "I need a holiday after my holiday!" is a commonly heard refrain. For most of us, it may have been a break from work, but not really a break. Celebrations over the holiday season are a time to connect with family and friends. There are a number of events planned, including dinners out with colleagues, and house parties with friends and neighbors that can go late into the night. There are family members, visiting us or whom we visit, that we do not see much during the rest of the year. There are the advance preparations of writing and sending greeting cards, and meal and menu planning, holiday baking, decorating the house. Then, there's the shopping—for groceries, for a new outfit for the parties, for gifts. Just thinking about it all again is exhausting! Regular reminders of why we choose to do all this help; we can recall what's good about this, and balance the work with the fun!

However, there are times when there is simply too much to do. How does one choose what to accept and what to decline? Balancing our lives is all about making choices. We need to choose things that we like to do, and from this list, choose only some of them. That means we have to choose to not do things we enjoy! This is the inherent challenge of achieving a balanced life—so difficult for us, as highly functioning individuals, because there is too much we like to do. We cannot do everything we want, not all at the same time.

If I had to redesign the human body (no, I'm not holding my breath waiting for the phone call from God!), the only thing that I would add is an Energy Gauge. I am reminded of an old Nintendo game my sons used to play years ago called Super Mario Brothers. In this game, Mario and his brother, Luigi, have to save the Princess Toadstool from an evil King Bowser, and have to conquer castles in eight different worlds in the Mushroom Kingdom to find and free the Princess. What really impressed me was how the characters were shown with these gauges on the top right hand corner of the screen that showed how much energy they had; how long they could continue to fight before they had to stop. Along the way, they move forward, find Power Up's that give them extra energy, and battle evil; their gauge shows progressively reduced levels of energy. At some point, even the young boys learned that they had to stop advancing and fighting, and just look for ways to replenish energy. I recall those pools into which Mario would sink, and his energy meter would just rise back to top levels so he could go off again. (Sinking into a full bathtub at the end of a long day reminds me of Mario's pool!)

We all should come with such a gauge. As we advance through our day, we could see just how much energy we are using up, and define that point when we stop advancing and look for ways to replenish our stores. This is when we stop accepting and start declining. We could even do this proactively, choosing advance limits, and not waiting to reach that endpoint. We do this regularly for our cars. The gas gauge adjusts as we use up gas, and as we get to near-empty (and hopefully before the warning light goes on), we veer off course to find a gas station to fill up.

The gas gauge analogy is a good one to keep in mind when we start another year. Hopefully, we are starting off with a full "tank" of energy, reenergized by our full but satisfying holiday season. Then, we can set a goal of maintaining our tanks above the halfway mark. This means two things: making sure we top it up, as well as limiting the drain out.

We can identify things that help us top up the tank, the equivalent of the gas station or Mario's pool, and proactively plan to include a stop there regularly in our day/week/year. This can be things like taking a quiet moment to ourselves, being with people that we enjoy, planning and taking short breaks and longer holidays, looking at pictures of loved ones, eating healthy foods, sleeping in on the weekends, watching a favorite movie, cuddling, exercising regularly, giving hugs to people we care about, learning something new, playing or listening to music, smiling, journaling, reading a great book, relaxing by the fireplace, meditating, laughing, luxuriating in a warm bath, buying flowers, sipping an afternoon tea.

We can also identify things that drain our tanks, including heavy workloads, stressful environments, packed schedules, too much responsibility, conflict and tension, and difficult interactions with demanding people. These will need to be limited and monitored carefully. In anticipation of these, we could plan things concomitantly that top up the tank to balance the drain.

Keeping the virtual energy gauge in mind, we need to consciously work to keep it (ideally) over the half-full mark all the time. Having built up a good reserve, we will have the ability, energy, enthusiasm, and confidence to go the distance.

SECTION THREE

Time Well Wasted

Many physicians do not actually look forward to a break. They think about being at home and not working, and feel guilty, and become anxious and unsettled. The unstructured time is most uncomfortable, and they just want to make lists to fill it up. This, however, leads to the family becoming upset or frustrated upset with them. "I wish that I were still at work or on call, so I would have an excuse to stay busy," one colleague confided.

Many physicians have difficulty taking time off and relaxing. Our personalities have been described by Gabbard, 1985, as a compulsive triad that includes doubt, guilt, and exaggerated sense of responsibility. Our insecurities and sense of responsibility drive us to work hard, and we feel very guilty if we do not meet this level of responsibility. This guilt actually makes us increase our professional activities, not decrease them.

Allowing time for leisure is not easy. Only about 10% of physicians take time off to relax and have real holidays. The rest of us either take holidays but do not really relax, combine it with a medical conference or course, or do not take time off.

The anxiety I describe is not uncommon among colleagues. Unstructured time often provokes this response, and I often hear that "it is easier to work than go on holidays." Many of us fill in this lack of structure with chores, projects, activities, and to-do lists. It is hard to "do nothing, to waste time." We need to be productive, to have "something to show for it."

Last year, there was a major unexpected power outage in Ontario and Eastern US. It took me by surprise, as at first, I did not know what to do. I headed to the computer about three times before I remembered that I could not check my emails. I could not cook the dinner I had planned. I could not turn on the television to find out what was happening. I could not even fill in the time and vacuum! Once I accepted this, we ended up having one of the most wonderful and memorable evenings of the year. We headed out into the street and organized a giant neighborhood barbecue from our freezers, and the kids freely enjoyed the ice cream and Popsicles, saved from melting. Our family ended the evening playing Scrabble by candlelight. I realized that we were not alone. As I spoke with neighbors and colleagues, I heard of the most wonderful stories of personal relaxation and connection with others that evening.

The Comedy Network on television has a wonderful slogan— "Time Well Wasted!" Let's make a New Year's resolution to learn to waste time well, without waiting for it to be forced upon us. Think of all the things we have managed to learn so far in our lives. We can learn this, too. This means learning to let our selves do nothing, identifying the associated anxiety, and balancing it with the fact that there is not need for this anxiety. We can reframe this "waste" of time, as an "investment" of time. As we take and invest time for ourselves, this allows us to reenergize and be more available to meet the needs of others who need us.

This means spending time in activities after which you will have nothing to show for it…like sitting back in bed, reading a book or magazine for fun, staying in your pyjamas all day, watching movies, lying in a hammock, watching the birds at the feeder, drinking a cup of tea until it's all finished, listening to music, playing, sleeping in. It means deciding that you will not check your emails or turn on your computer. It means pretending that the stores are not open on Sundays. It means enjoying the moment you are in, and relishing the time with your family and friends, giving them your full attention.

Practice makes perfect. The more of this you do, the easier it gets. Once you get the hang of it, use the Tarzan Rule to keep it going. Just as Tarzan swings through the jungle and does not let go of the rope until he has the next one in hand, don't end a relaxing break, without having booked the next one. Enjoy your holiday.

Women in Medicine

As our medical schools are opening their door to more women than ever before, they are also opening the door to change. In the past few decades, increasing numbers of women have been entering medical school. In recent years, there are actually more women than men in Canadian medical school classes. I have heard colleagues from medical schools and organizations say that there is no longer a need for gender-focused committees, as there are no longer any issues about women in medicine. I disagree, and believe that the issues are not resolved but have changed, from supporting more women getting into medicine, to addressing how they can succeed and be supported in how they practice medicine. There is no doubt that women practice medicine differently than their male colleagues, and that this will impact on health care.

There are a few key studies that have investigated the impact of increased numbers of women in medicine. This increase was already being noted over 30 years ago, by Dr. Naomi Bluestone, in her 1978 paper in the American Journal of Public Health on the impact of women physicians on American medicine. She described how women physicians had been known in the past to favor the three P's—pediatrics, public health, and psychiatry; often did not marry; made less money than their male colleagues; and had not risen in the medical academic ranks. She wrote about significant changes occurring which showed more women choosing to enter medicine, working longer hours, being more insistent upon recompense, and moving into more varied disciplines including surgery. She commented on how women practiced medicine differently—tending to work better with other women health professionals, more empathic and intuitive, more vocal in protecting themselves from prejudices, and establishing more mutually supportive networks. Yet, while they were not ready to sacrifice family and outside interests for their career, they were also not ready to accept a second-class career. In doing so, they caused male colleagues to question their own attitudes, and lifestyle choices, and seek similar flexibility.

OPTIMIZE TRAINING TO PRODUCE RESULTS

In 1990, a Canadian Medical Association Journal article by Williams et al, described how female physicians bring distinctive values that are reflected in how they conduct their professional practices. Women tended to prefer group over solo practice, only one third were in medical specialties, were working fewer hours than men, and even after adjusting for differences in workloads, their incomes were significantly lower than those of the men.

The Changing Face of Medicine by Boulis and Jacobs, 2008, looks at why more women are entering medicine, how they are faring personally and professionally, and how they are transforming medicine. The material draws on multiple sources, including interviews with women physicians. They describe how women's roles in contemporary society, not just in medicine, have changed. Women physicians' families are becoming more and more like those of other working women. Yet, there are still gender disparities in terms of specialty, practice ownership, academic rank, leadership roles, and limits to opportunity.

The Royal College of Physicians in the United Kingdom recently released a study on the increasing number of women in medical schools, and how they are set to overtake men in many areas of medicine within a decade. However, women seem to be more likely to opt for specialties with "plannable" working hours, work part-time, and are less represented among top medical leaders. This may mean that these specific specialties could face shortages. The report highlights the need to adapt to this situation to maintain high standards in medicine, summarizes the organizational implications of this trend, and offers recommendations for policymakers to address future issues of medical workforce and its design.

I have personally witnessed the same change in colleagues through my practice over the past twenty years. There are more women in medicine, and nearly half of medical students are now female. Women are making patient care friendlier, spend more time in patient care, form stronger bonds with their patients, and are less likely to be sued. Women are more likely to go into primary care, and serve minority and needier populations. Women are more likely to shoulder the bulk of family and home responsibilities, want to balance work and home life, and so work fewer hours than male colleagues and focus less on achieving leadership roles. The reality is that career building and family building occur during the same years.

This does have implications for the medical workforce, along with other factors such as aging and retirement of the current medical workforce, and an aging population. This will lead to a shortfall and require health human resource planning to account for this. There will need to be increased numbers of doctors to be trained, encouragement of physicians to go into specialties currently less likely to be chosen by women, and looking at how these specialities can be more compatible with better work/life balance.

Yet, an increase in the number of women in medicine has led to improvements in medicine, too. Women physicians have helped to make it more acceptable for both men and women to choose to achieve a healthy balance between work and home lives. They serve as agents for primary prevention and personal health promotion. A colleague told me about how he was denied permission to leave to attend the delivery of his first child, 25 years ago. Men now have the opportunity for paternity leave, to leave the OR to pick up their children from daycare, and to refuse extra work if personal and family plans have already been made. As a result, perhaps we may see more doctors avoiding burnout, and enjoying work. Patients like seeing a doctor who is energetic, enjoying their work, and happy to be there, and thereby more likely to sustain a long term practice. Healthy doctors are good role models for patients. We know that a healthy doctor leads to a healthier community.

OPTIMIZE TRAINING TO PRODUCE RESULTS

Reluctant Leaders: Women Physicians as Leaders

There are more Physician Leadership Conferences available than ever before. As a busy woman physician, I often found myself in leadership positions, without much formal leadership training. We are all capable of learning on the job, especially with great mentors and supporters, yet it is wonderful to have opportunities to reflect and learn.

One does not have to hold an administrative title or position to be a leader. Every physician is a leader. A leader is someone who has talent and specific skills, initiative and drive, charismatic inspiration and is liked by others and serves to motivate them, dedicates their life to a cause, has a clear sense of mission with focus and commitment, is results oriented, optimistic and determined, and serves as a role model. We show all of these skills on a daily basis, when we see patients; teach students; carry out research; chair committees; run clinics, departments, and hospitals; coach Little League baseball; or volunteer in our community. Many physicians are Reluctant Leaders—they did not seek to be a leader, rather saw a need for a change or improvement and took it on because it had some meaning for them.

We are lucky in Canada to have access to several excellent medical leadership courses through the Canadian Medical Association, and well as leadership conferences in conjunction with the Canadian Society of Physician Executives. The Physician Manager Institute (PMI) offers more advanced leadership and management skills, aimed at physicians having or considering management responsibilities. It addresses topics such as performance management, managing people, managing conflicts, negotiation process, change process, communication, team building skills, and problem solving skills. Physicians in other countries also have access to excellent leadership workshops and courses.

Leadership can be passive or leading by example, where one starts from within, showing traits that others want to emulate, and resulting in others being inspired by, and following, a leader.

There is Active Leadership, when one wants change and makes a conscious decision to lead to it. These are not separate and distinct, and there is a continuum of both of these types of leadership styles, where one can evolve into the other. People can lead with formal authority, informal authority, or even no authority (you just need the will, not the position). Interestingly, many women lead successfully without formal authority. Women physicians need to give themselves credit for the leadership roles they have taken, and to move ahead on an issue in which they believe.

Dianne Buckner, of CBC News World's Venture, once spoke about the *Seven Things that Women Are Not Told About Leadership*. These were:

7. The rules for men and women are different. Men are applauded and respected for being aggressive and frank, women are criticized for this.

6. Important decisions are often made informally. This can include times such as during a golf game, and may exclude women.

5. Check your ovaries at the door. It is known that women without children are more likely to be promoted, that as many as 40% of female executives do not plan to have children, and even when family-friendly policies exist, women are hesitant to use them.

4. Success in leadership does not mean that you are a genius. Good ideas can come easily; it is the ability to implement them that matters. Show integrity and follow through on your ideas.

3. Women should be better at promoting themselves. Women often remain modest and shy, and minimize or even dismiss their achievements.

2. Women are instinctive leaders. They are mothers naturally, and lead and direct families. It's in our nature.

OPTIMIZE TRAINING TO PRODUCE RESULTS

1. Being a leader can be uncomfortable at times. Expect it to be bumpy, and be confident that you can ride it out.

Hearing such words of wisdom, and gaining such specific skills, is a unique experience not found elsewhere in our medical training and continuing education. I hope this will give you a taste of what you can gain, and whet your appetite for more, to become the leader you can be.

SECTION FOUR

BUILDING HIGH PERFORMANCE TEAMS: HEALTHY MEDICAL WORKPLACES

SECTION FOUR

Physician Morale & Burnout

Physician morale seems to be at an all-time low. Morale is a key ingredient of a successful workplace. According to the American Heritage Dictionary, morale is the state of the spirits of a person or group, as exhibited by confidence, cheerfulness, discipline, willingness to perform assigned tasks, and dedication to a common cause. While doctors, as a group, are known to be dedicated, hard-working, conscientious, and wanting to please others, many are finding it increasingly difficult to maintain a positive outlook. In my practice, colleagues constantly tell me that they would accept that they are working harder than ever before, with fewer resources, if only they felt it was worth it in terms of better patient care. Yet, most of the time they feel that despite greater efforts, they are still not providing the level of patient care they would like.

A colleague told me that each day that he goes into work at the medical clinic, he is struck by how things have steadily declined. Physician morale seems low. People seem to be unhappy, impatient, irritable, and are starting to keep to themselves. He chose to work in this clinic over a solo practice, so that he would not be lonely. Is it possible to feel lonely with others around?

Morale is related to burnout. Burnout is a state of chronic stress due to workplace problems, in which people become negative, feel they are being acted upon and not exercising choice, and start to pull away from colleagues and lose a sense of job satisfaction. The pulling away from others is, indeed, very isolating. It is not possible to maintain good morale in this situation.

I know that even the strongest and healthiest of physicians are capable of becoming ill in an unhealthy environment. According to the Canadian Centre for Occupational Health and Safety (1999), an unhealthy workplace can triple the chance of cardio-vascular disease, double the chance of substance abuse, and increase injuries, infections, and mental illness. A 2002 discussion paper from the Canadian Policy Research Networks shows that health professionals are the least likely of all workers to describe their work environment as healthy, with job satisfaction below the national average.

The workplace environment is made up of structural and psychosocial aspects. A good environment allows for trust, sense of belonging and commitment, and a feeling of being appreciated. Problems arise when there is a mismatch between the person doing the job and what the job requires in terms of any or all of the following areas: workload, sense of control and choice, reward and recognition, community and connection, fairness and respect, ability to meet own values.

The workload for physicians is higher than ever before. There are more treatments and procedures possible; more things that we can offer a patient now. Patients are living longer and requiring more intervention. Families are having fewer children and the expectation of health is greater than ever before. There are financial cutbacks and limitations, and so fewer physicians are present to share the workload. Newer graduates in medicine want to have a more balanced life, and so often are not taking the same share of the workload as their senior colleagues. Work expectations and priorities need to be clearly defined. The resources that are available to get the work done must be highlighted, and efforts made to create further resources. Time for reflection of your work is helpful, where you can take time to consider and look for ways to optimize the situation. Physicians can learn to say no, and set limits. They also need to learn to accept when a colleague says no, respecting and understanding how hard it is to do so.

There is a sense of lack of control and choice over issues at work. This needs to be acknowledged openly. It helps to address this openly, and identify as a group what things you can and cannot control. While you may not be able to control that people get sick, need care often urgently, that we have limited resources, and yet need to earn an income; you can control some aspects such as what you have available to care for patients, how you work together, how you pool income, and how much you work.

SECTION FOUR

Colleagues are encouraged to support each other to cope with things that are not under your control, and to share strategies for dealing with these issues.

As humans, we need to feel appreciated for what we do. The medical workplace is not known for constant praise and encouragement. There is a distinct sense of lack of reward and recognition. As a group, you can explore ways to make someone feel appreciated, and encourage doing this more often. It helps to understand why this is difficult to do, and identify strategies to make it easier. Positive reinforcement should be immediate and specific. Some ideas include saying thank you, writing a short thank you note on a post-it note and sticking it to their door, thank you cards, celebrating birthdays and special events as a group, sending flowers or small gifts. In your clinic, consider setting up a bulletin board to post achievements, creating an "unsung hero" award, or putting together a small newsletter with positive stories of the clinic activities and the people in it. In Ottawa, the medical community has worked with the mayor to proclaim a day in October as Physician Appreciation Day. The goal is to expand this throughout the province and country in the coming years.

Being busier than ever before, we may not have the time to promote a sense of community and connection in our workplace. We are too busy to take the time to get together to eat lunch, or go for a walk. Computers have made communication easier, yet more remote. It is now easier and quicker to send off a quick email than to take the time to seek out a colleague to talk with them. Thus, we feel increasingly isolated. Medical workplaces can find ways to communicate in person, stay connected, and work as a group. Senior colleagues can take a mentoring role, and lead the fostering of a sense of team, and help newcomers get oriented and incorporated into the group. A retreat, or team building exercise, is helpful and fun. Try finding out interesting things about a colleague that you did not know before. Relate to them as people, not just someone with whom you work. The concept of an Emotional Bank Account is excellent. It involves assuming that consistent efforts made within a relationship with each colleague are like deposits to a bank, and making regular deposits consciously. When you are upset, you will make a "withdrawal" but, hopefully, will still have a positive balance left. Try to set up such a "bank" with each of your colleagues! Think good will. Group communication is an area worthy of regular review. Workshops on conflict management, learning to identify needs, listen to each other, and negotiate compromises are successful in helping to deal with difficult situations.

Some groups suffer from a lack of fairness, and respect for each other's contributions. It is best when your group can address this, and accept that the value of work is dependent on the time it takes to do it. That is, an hour of clinical work is as valuable as administrative work, teaching, or research. Encourage a mix of focus, and a chance to try out another type of work, so one can best appreciate what a colleague does.

Tension at work can occur if there is a conflict of values. Colleagues in your workplace must be given the opportunity to express concerns and differences of opinions, and be listened to, and offered empathy.

All of these areas take time to address. The ideal way is to have a retreat, where these issues and goals to address them can be raised. This must be followed by regular ongoing assessments, to maintain the relationships and priorities. Taking time to listen to each other, understand how things are for them, connect, and express appreciation and value is the best way to connect, and thus restore physician morale.

Compassion in Medical Workplace

I was speaking to a younger colleague last week who stopped me in the hall to thank me. She had just taken on a position as her department's residency Program Director, and was really enjoying it. As I spoke to her, she described other initiatives she had recently taken on within the department. She was enthusiastic and full of energy. Her youngest child had just started junior kindergarten and "normal life had begun again."

She expressed her gratitude and admiration for how her Department Chair had supported her during the past several years. While she was a resident, he had recognized her potential, and offered her a job upon completion of her fellowship. He was gracious and congratulatory when she announced each of her pregnancies, and allowed her to adjust her workload and call schedules as required. The department had sent her flowers and gifts when the babies were born, and she was told to enjoy her maternity leave and not rush back. When she returned, she was able to work part time to accommodate her family's busy schedule. She told me that her Department Chair had been so wonderfully supportive, and that she was forever grateful, and happy to pay back now. "They have invested so much in me; I will do all I can now and be the best attending they have ever had." She was committed and dedicated to her department, and ready to realize the potential they had seen in her.

She told me she was thanking me because her Chair had confided to her that he had made a concerted effort to be more supportive after hearing me talk about the benefits of this strategy at a department chair retreat. He recalled that I had encouraged them all to support the junior members of the department for a few years, and reassured them that they would, in turn, get back the most dedicated hard-working colleague forever.

I thought back to my own experience. I was finishing my fellowship, had three babies—a year old son, and newborn twins—and was exploring job options. I had asked my department chair if I could work part-time, but he said that all he could offer was a fulltime job, "Take it or leave it." Unable to meet the requirements for call, I had to turn down the position, and went into private practice. I often reflect on what I could have done as a more active part of the department. I was pleased that this colleague had such a different experience from mine, and thus had such a deep sense of belonging and commitment to her department.

Compassion in the workplace is an integral factor leading to improved morale and satisfaction and productivity. It occurs when one notices the pain or need of another, feels empathy, and reaches out and responds. There is big and lasting impact of small acts of kindness and thoughtfulness. The recipient appreciates this, feels a sense of belonging, and is motivated to pay it forward. Compassion matters, and leads to increased retention, improved work satisfaction, and commitment.

The value of compassion in the workplace was largely anecdotal until recently. Dr. Jacoba Lilius, of the School of Policy Studies, at Queen's University, heads a Compassion Lab, where she and her colleagues have explored core questions about compassion at work. Their work indicates that compassion occurs with relative frequency, and suggests a relationship between experienced compassion, positive emotion, and affective commitment, thereby providing evidence of the powerful consequences of compassion.

Medical clinics, departments, hospitals, and other organizations can work to enable compassion in their work environment. People are, in fact, predisposed to want this, and to respond to it. Workplace leaders can encourage or stifle it. A small effort into encouraging compassion among your group, with formal policies that support workers, setting healthy norms, highlighting examples, and role modelling such behaviour, will lead to lasting positive impact.

SECTION FOUR

Dealing with Difficult Behaviour

It is wonderful to see that physician health is becoming more of a recognized issue in our current health care environment. I am gratified to see how much support and energy and momentum this concept has gained in the past 10 years. Initial work focused on improving the personal health of colleagues, and this continued to include advocating for a healthy medical workplace.

One of the key factors in ensuring a healthy workplace in medicine is to provide a safe and supportive collegial environment. This has led to increasing awareness of disruptive behaviour. Commonsense tells us that it exists but the literature is just emerging and sparse. Disruptive behaviour is defined as poor communication behaviours, including intimidation, which cause negative impact on others in the workplace. There is usually a longstanding history; it often goes on for years unaddressed. It is rarely one isolated incident; rather multiple similar reports from a variety of sources.

There are three main types of inappropriate behaviours, as identified by Irons, in 1994:

Inappropriate Anger includes sudden and unpredictable outbursts, rude or abusive conduct to staff, patients, and patients' families, yelling, and intimidation.

Inappropriate Response includes verbal attacks of staff which can be personal, unfair, public; non-constructive criticism and belittling, unnecessary sarcasm or cynicism, profane or disrespectful language, blaming others, sexual innuendos, and slurs.

Inappropriate Action includes sexual harassment, late or unsuitable responses to pages, imposing unreasonable expectations and demands on staff, throwing objects, and bullying.

There are many contributing factors, including stress and burnout, especially later stages; substance abuse, medical diseases, and psychiatric disorders such as depression, anxiety, mania, dementia, OCD, and personality disorders.

This behaviour is unacceptable and needs to be addressed. It can have negative impact on the health of the physician, and his/her family; negative impact on other heath care professionals who work with them and may feel job dissatisfaction, reduced morale, helplessness, tension, and anxiety; negative impact on patient care; and impact on the overall medical organization.

However, it is not easy to address such behaviour. It makes us feel uncomfortable and tense. It is easier to avoid conflict. We may feel disloyal to the colleague, as if we are "tattling." We worry that we won't be believed, have no power, or will have the burden of proof; and risk liability and reprisal. Often, if this is longstanding behaviour, such people are charming, high achievers, successful, and in senior positions.

The typical response of medical colleagues who are intelligent, nice, caring, and understanding is to deny (let it go), minimize (look the other way), or rationalize (hope it is temporary and will stop). They avoid any direct discussion, but eventually, they become frustrated and resentful, and this can lead to a confrontation.

To encourage and support reporting of such behaviour, many medical organizations have adopted a zero tolerance policy for such behaviour violations. This is a great step forward overall.

However, there is a pattern that I have seen emerging in recent years among colleagues working in a small or rural community, in a health care system with decreasing resources. These colleagues are dedicated and conscientious physicians, who work hard to establish their practices, provide excellent patient care, make themselves available, and soon shoulder a very heavy workload. As demands increase, they feel unable to say "No" and set limits. Often, there are few other resources, they may be doing 1-in-2 call, they may be the only ones who can do a specific procedure—so they agree to do more with the justification that the ultimate goal is to provide the best patient care. However, this is not sustainable. These colleagues ask for help, but it is not available. They are tired, become resentful, have an angry outburst, and then are identified as "disruptive doctors."

While they do have disruptive behaviour, they are not truly disruptive doctors.

I fully support the recent increased awareness of such behaviour as inappropriate and unacceptable. However, the response to such situations needs to be to explore and assess the situation thoroughly. There are many causes of such behaviour, each of which requires different solutions. In the situation described above, such labelling is not only inaccurate, but unhelpful, as it can prevent a successful resolution.

In fact, the colleagues in this situation are experiencing burnout due to chronic work stress and high workloads. They are a victim of their own success, as they initially set a pace that was not sustainable. They do not have a psychiatric diagnosis or a personality disorder. *Any highly functioning healthy person placed in an unhealthy situation can become unhealthy.* None of us are immune. While they do need to learn to gain insight into their need for approval and difficulty in limit-setting, and learn to assert their needs in a calm and professional manner, it is also essential that the institution understand their vulnerability to burnout, express appreciation of their work, and actively support them with the needed resources to maintain a healthy and sustainable work-life balance. Ideal resolution can only be achieved by fully addressing both aspects of this situation.

Medical organizations can ideally establish a policy for dealing with such behaviour, institute it, and publish it. This will outline a clear and transparent procedure to deal with such a colleague, in a written policy outlining explicit expectations and zero tolerance. It should include early identification of such behaviour, clear documentation of all incidents and trends, constructive feedback, education of the physician, and a fair and confidential reporting process. The first response to such reports would be to approach the physician in a safe and confidential manner, confront the behaviour clearly and firmly and specifically, and provide them a chance to explain and clear it up. There can be arrangements for clinical assessments, options provided for therapy and gaining skills, with clear consequences of continued negative behaviour. This will require regular monitoring and follow-up evaluations.

The workplace itself will need to be accountable, and offer confirmation that they are providing an optimal workplace. I recognize that this may be especially true for rural settings, where physicians have fewer resources. The ideal administration would be supportive of physician's health needs, be alert to early warning signs of stress and burnout, and allow any required workplace accommodations. An initial orientation workshop for new doctors in the community could be created to define roles and expectations, understanding and avoiding burnout, effective communication skills, assertive training, and conflict resolution skills. All incidents need to be identified and addressed early. Prompt assistance from workplace mediators and counsellors could avoid later resentments, complaints, lawsuits, or dismissals.

Only by addressing both the unprofessional behaviour and improving a suboptimal workplace environment, will successful resolution be fully achieved.

Teamwork: Collaborative Health Care

I am just returning from a conference on collaborative practices in health care, which brought together over 800 doctors, nurses, and pharmacists to explore ways in which we can collaborate to improve health care. It got me thinking more about this development in health care, and how it will be part of the new landscape of how we practice medicine in Canada. The medical news is full of such developments—pharmacists assuming the authority to prescribe medications in defined situations, nurse anaesthesia assistants, and family health teams. There is a lot of discussion, resistance, and defensiveness.

In 2003, Health Canada defined a Collaborative Patient-Centered Practice as one that is designed to promote the active participation of several health care disciplines and professions. It would enhance patient, family, and community centered goals and values, provide mechanisms for continuous communication among health care providers, optimize staff participation in clinical decision making within and across disciplines, and foster respect for the contributions of all providers.

While this sounds wonderful in theory, there are many barriers to collaborative care in medicine. There is a common history and similar goals of patient care; yet each discipline has a different culture, training, and education, and so addresses issues from differing points of view.

As doctors, our personality traits can hinder collaboration. We are conscientious and perfectionistic, and so can be rigid and inflexible. We have a need to be in control, and so have difficulty delegating to others, or changing how we have done things in the past. Our sense of responsibility makes it hard to let others do things that we feel are ultimately ours to do. Our ability to delay gratification allows us to work until it is all done, yet makes us more prone to being tired, irritable, and impatient—characteristics that do not endear us to our health care colleagues. At times, we feel insecure and need to do more; we micromanage to help us feel more reassured and confident. These uncertainties can add to our concerns about blurring of roles and responsibilities, "turf wars," how we will be financially reimbursed, possible loss of our jobs, negative impact on patient safety and care. Additionally, this new way of practice requires training and education and time, when time is always at a premium.

I wonder if some of this uncertainty results from our experiences in an earlier type of collaboration—that between doctors and midwives. This had a turbulent start, as midwives were seen as anti-doctor, and took control of a birth situation, often outside of a hospital with little resources available, and only called the doctor when there was serious trouble. Outcomes were poor, and doctors were often involved in lawsuits and complaints. Who wants to come into a clinical situation in a crisis? The reality is that this was uncommon, and when it occurred it was not really collaboration—rather two professions working independently. Better examples of collaboration would be case room nurses and doctors, and how doctors and midwives have learned to work comfortably with each other, communicate well, know and respect their own and others limitations, and ask for help.

Regardless of how we feel about this, collaboration in medicine is happening, and may well be "the way we do things" in the near future. We may as well be proactive, and help shape this into a positive situation. This is a change, and while no one likes change, it is usually necessary and productive. It is essential to include people in the process, get input so one has buy in, set mutual goals, and identify champions of change within the system. It is harder to make a change and enforce it after the fact—a situation I see is occurring now that the Ontario Ministry of Health announced the creation of anaesthesia care teams recently to reduce wait times, but did not appropriately include the anaesthesiologists in this decision-making process

It helps to remember what is good about collaboration. There are now fewer resources in medicine, with less manpower and cutbacks. There are more women in medicine, and a younger generation, both groups who practice differently with more regard to a healthier balanced lifestyle. Thus, they are not willing to work the long hours of a senior generation of doctors. Working with other health care professionals with increased scope of duties may prevent provider burnout, offer assistance, free up time for doctors, and allow increased access to appropriate, timely care for patients.

Working in a team does not mean that one is engaging in teamwork. Teams work well with attention to seven key aspects:

- Clear goals and purpose.
- Clear roles and responsibilities.
- Clear and regular communication.
- Mutual respect and trust.
- Defined processes for tasks.
- Effective leadership.
- Effective organizational structure with regular meetings, preferably face-to-face.

Thus, there is a need for education on all of these areas. All members of the health care team will benefit from specific training as a team. This can assist in setting and clarifying roles and responsibilities, and providing reassurance that this is not substitution but a realignment of the system to make it work better. Doctors are usually relieved to know that they are not legally responsible for the clinical work of another regulated health professional. On a team, they are only directly legally responsible for their own clinical work and patient care, for communicating about patients as they hand over care, and for enforcing policies and procedures if they are an administrative leader. While teams need leaders, and doctors are not the only ones who can lead, doctors do make effective leaders as it is a role in which they often have training, comfort, and experience. A team leader can play a key role in the facilitation of recognition of the value of all team members. Trust within a medical team is built as one profession can see and value what the other is doing to provide better care to the patient. We all feel a personal responsibility to our patient and cannot hand him over to just anyone. Regular communication is crucial, especially in the early stages of setting up a team. This communication needs to be open and direct and timely.

As doctors, we have all the skills to make a team work. It is crucial to approach this with an open attitude, and remember that we are all working on the same team and have a common goal of providing the best possible care to our patients. Many doctors say that once they have worked on a team, they cannot imagine how they ever did it without the team, and that they would never go back to the old way.

Our current problems are a result of our past successes; we have created overwhelming confidence and expectations and demands from our patients because we have done such a great job to date. Collaborative care allows us to add support to an overburdened system, and to share energies, ethics, values, and concerns to meet the increasing needs of patients.

SECTION FOUR

Learning Among the Generations

Many mid-career physicians have been noticing that younger medical colleagues seem to have a different attitude towards medicine. They seem to be better at setting limits and meeting their own needs. At times, older colleagues feel cynical and critical of this, and become frustrated and resentful, especially when these younger ones want to have responsibilities and positions without putting in the time to earn them. Other times, they feel envious and inspired to do the same.

There is no doubt that the impact of Generation X is being felt within medicine, as in all other aspects of society. There is a generational shift as the workforce ages, and younger colleagues enter and change the face of the work environment. How can we better understand, and work productively and professionally with them?

While definitions vary, Generation X is a term that generally refers to those born after the Baby Boomers, between 1961 and 1981. This group makes up roughly a third of the workforce. Many authors have described common traits within this group. They are confident, questioning, challenging, and individualistic. They have a high degree of comfort and knowledge with technology. Their focus is on balancing their lifestyles, and having time for themselves and their family. They are not as motivated by, or awed by, income and status as previous generations. They view the older generation as being too rigid and demanding.

In the medical workplace, this attitude can easily be misinterpreted as being less caring, less committed, less dedicated, less respectful. Senior colleagues have devoted themselves to medicine, at times at the expense of their family or themselves. This was seen as the normal standard. I recall a general surgeon who taught me as an intern. Of the 1-in-2 call on his rotation, he told the team "It's a shame; you will be missing half of what you need to see." Recently, a colleague spoke to me of wanting to slow down and retire in coming years. He had been working in a small town for 40 years, five long days each week, and hoped to recruit a new doctor to the town so he could cut down to four days a week, He was stunned to hear that while this junior colleague was interested in working with him, he wanted to start at three days a week.

It helps to understand this younger generation by reviewing what they experienced growing up. Born after the Women's Liberation Movement, most of them had two working parents. They saw firsthand the impact on the family, the lack of time for the children, the high levels of stress and burnout. The "standard" was recognized as imperfect. Their reaction was to vow to not do the same, to work less and not allow this to happen.

This group is seen as impatient and entitled. They want to get responsibilities and positions, without putting in the time, or respecting what it took others to achieve this. I was speaking to a junior colleague a few years ago, and telling him how I had advocated hard on his behalf to offer him a largely responsible position despite his inexperience, because of his interest and enthusiasm and potential. I suppose I expected that he would be appreciative (of my work on his behalf), but also gain an awareness of this situation and tread cautiously with senior colleagues in a grateful and respectful manner. Instead of appreciation and understanding, he stated "I hate that ageism."

Again, this sense of entitlement to, and expectation of, responsibilities can be understood in context. These were the Latch-Key Kids. They often came home to an empty house, had the responsibility of having their own key and letting themselves in, perhaps preparing their own snack, organizing their own activities, starting their own homework. This group was given responsibilities at an early age—they took it and rose to the task.

They anticipate similar levels of responsibility in the work-place, and feel they have shown they can do it. In fact, they are skilled at this, and do have much to offer. Instead of resenting or blocking this, it can be much more productive to assess their skills and strengths, and plan to give them responsibilities, starting with smaller roles and titles.

SECTION FOUR

While much of the focus is on the Generation X'ers in medicine, there are in fact four generations now working side-by-side within the medical workplace. There are the older Veterans, the Baby Boomers, Generation X, and Generation Y (born after 1981). Understanding, accepting, and embracing the generational differences will assist in these groups working together. They all have different and complementary strengths, and can work effectively together.

There are some positive and effective strategies for senior physicians to foster improved relationships among the generations:

- Understand each others differences, without judgment or criticism.

- Identify each others strengths.

- Offer Improved mentoring of the younger groups, especially in aspects of leadership and skills development.

- Promote flexibility to allow healthier work-life balance, respect and support their needs and values.

- Offer small roles and responsibilities to junior colleagues, with clear goals and deadlines. Do not "baby" them; this is seen as condescending.

- Allow them independence in planning for and reaching the goals. Do not micromanage.

- Support their ideas. Encourage their opinions, and listen to them.

- Foster creativity, thinking "outside the box," and positive change.

- Provide constructive, timely, clear feedback.

- Foster networks and connections within teams, and with other colleagues.

The culture of medicine is changing, with changing attitudes, values, and norms from new generations of physician. This is the future; it is not going to go away. While slow and difficult, change is generally positive and healthy. We need to embrace and work with it, not fear and resist this. While how things were done in the past did work, a new way can work well, too. The title of an excellent book on managing change by Kriegel and Brandt summarizes this best; *Sacred Cows Make the Best Burgers.*

SECTION FIVE

STRENGTH TRAINING AFTER INJURY: TRANSITIONS IN LIFE

SECTION FIVE

Being Single

I have just returned from a weekend out of town at a conference. While the days were busy, long and full, I returned each evening to the beautifully appointed hotel room alone. I appreciated the sound of silence, and the awareness that things were just as I had left them (okay, not really, they were cleaner!). It was such a treat to be in control of the television remote, and watch whatever I wanted. At home, there is no way that the boys would ever let me watch "What Not To Wear" when sports are always available on another channel. Finally, I stretched out and luxuriated on the huge bed, revelling in having all four pillows to myself. The assumption is that singles get to live like this all the time, relax when they want, yet live an exciting, joyful life, happily meeting all their needs, working hard to succeed, taking exotic holidays, driving fancy cars, going to fabulous parties, and having more money and freedom than they know what to do with. Wouldn't this be great all the time?

In fact, no it isn't. Many single doctors would prefer not to be single. (I did try to get some statistics on how many single doctors there are in Canada, but Google directed me to some very interesting sites that did not have this information, but did contain the words "single," and "doctor" as well as others such as sexy and dating—but I digress.) Let's accept that there are many single doctors—some never committed, some separated or divorced, and some widowed. Often, they tell me stories of being alone, but lonely and solitary—especially when one is suddenly left alone. They go home and are shocked by the silence, and wish there was something to do, and someone to do it with. Barbara Holland, in her book, *One's Company*, states "No doubt about it, solitude is improved by being voluntary."

It is not easy for a doctor who is single to find a partner. People assume that they are busy and not available, and do not invite them to events. If one lives in a small town, the list of those who are not patients and, therefore, possible options, is extremely narrow. The lifestyle is often too busy or hectic, leaving little time to meet people and pursue relationships. Patients tell me that there are now good ways to meet people that take less time. There are evenings of spin dating where one gets to meet can meet about 20 people in a single evening, talk to them for a short period of time, and can get contact information for any one would like to see again, if they had indicated that they would like to contact the other again, too. Online dating sites are now very acceptable and attractive to the busy professional, again allowing the chance to meet a lot of people with little investment of time. In larger cities, services such as *It's Just Lunch* focus on bringing together two busy professionals.

No amount of wishing will change the single's situation. It helps to identify what part one can control and focus on that. The first step is to stop waiting for it to change, and find a way to settle into it, for now, and make it comfortable. I recall when I first arrived at university and saw the tiny room in residence that I would call home for the coming year. Some of us on the residence floor did nothing to our room, spent as little time in it as possible, and complained about how awful it was. Yet, I recall a friend down the hall whose room we all hung out in. She had hung up some posters, put up her own curtains, and a matching bedspread, and bought a soft rug. We all spent the same time there at the dorm, but she did it more comfortably, enjoyed it, and was actually rarely alone. The ironic part is that the one who seems content in being on his own rarely is left to be alone.

Look proactively for what's good about being alone every day. Identify areas of interest that you have not had the chance to pursue and do so now. Take a class and learn something new. Join a group that focuses on the activity or area of interest that you enjoy. Think about what other people would want time alone to do, and do that—shop, read, go to the spa, watch TV or a movie, do nothing.

Make choices, keep busy.

Friends are an anchor for the single. Sure, couples have friends, but they don't need them the same way and the friendship often does not reach the same depth. Single adults need their friends. There are many different kinds of friends, and we need them all—the ones who support us emotionally, the ones who are direct and push us to do more, the fun ones, the ones who keep us young, the ones who inspire and mentor us. For some, single friends are ideal since they can have the same needs. One just needs to watch and ensure they are not too needy or draining. It is easier for those who are extroverted to make friends, and perhaps easier for women than men. Gather your friends around you; throw a party. Use the Tarzan Rule (don't end a fun event without planning the next one) to keep these contacts going.

Pets are great for company and unconditional love. They are constantly there, and come running when you arrive home, jumping up to you to give a lick. They don't care if you're having a bad hair day. All they want is that you know how to operate a can opener—a small requirement for big payoff! While some doctors feel they are too busy to have a pet, in fact, the pet and the care it requires serve to slow the pace of their life down to a sustainable level.

Family—parents and siblings—can be a big source of support for the single person. As with friends, the main thing for doctors is learning how to let others help them. They see their role as taking care of others, and may find it hard to be on the receiving end. Children in the home greatly assist in keeping one busy and full of a send of purpose. Yet, sadly they leave—just as they are becoming less work and more fun. Don't worry—they may be back!

Work is great. It gives structure to your life, earns money, and is a place where one can interact intimately with people. However, it can overtake one too easily. There is always more to be done, and the single doctor can feel guilty and responsible enough to stay longer and do more. Sometimes, the single doctor is asked to do more, on the assumption that they do not have to go home to a family. It helps to set limits in advance, remember that you have a life too, and that a healthy work/life balance is best.

Take care of yourself. It is not easy to cook interesting foods for yourself, yet that does not mean it is not possible. You are worth it! KD (Kraft Dinner) again is not acceptable. Pretend that your best friend is coming over for dinner—what would you make? Enjoy it for two days on your own. Make time to exercise and stay fit. Laugh. Reach out and get therapy if you feel it may help you understand and accept the situation.

Keep yourself open to meeting and loving.

SECTION FIVE

Moving to a New City

My resident is just finishing her residency and moving to a new city to start a practice. She is understandably nervous about starting in a new place, meeting people, and making friends. I remember feeling like this when I moved after medical school to start my residency in another place.

Transition is never easy. This one that she is about to make is even harder than most, as there are many changes all at once—a new job, new responsibilities, and a new place, where she does not know anyone yet.

Change is hectic, and stressful. Yet, it can also be exciting and full of opportunity. In this situation, it helps to remember you are not alone; apparently one in five families moves every year, and manages to survive it!

Organization is a key factor to a successful move. Lets break it down into phases of Before, During and After the move.

Before the Move:

Make a list of factors you need to consider and address, which can include:

Your stuff; sort through your belongings, pare down, give away items you do not need.

The move; do it yourself vs. movers. Do comparison shopping. Book it.

Change of address; to family and friends, at the bank, magazines, credit card companies, investment firms, professionals, organizations, motor vehicle bureau. Ask the post office to redirect your mail.

Banking; close or transfer accounts to new location.

Insurance; reassess how your needs will change with increased income or new possessions and responsibilities.

Utilities; organize cut-off dates, and arrange to start in new home before you arrive there.

Medical records; obtain from family doctor, dentist, vet, and arrange to have sent to new doctors.

Delivery services; discontinue delivery of newspapers, milk, diapers.

Clean out fridge and freezer; Stop buying groceries, and use up as much as you can. Give to friends, family, food banks.

Keep records of your moving expenses. You may be able to deduct these expenses, on your income tax return.

During the Move:

On moving day, it helps to carry with you:

- A small case with change of clothing and personal toiletry items.
- Medications.
- Cash or travelers' cheques.
- Jewellery.
- Important documents like house sale papers, important personal records.
- Phone numbers of moving company, insurance agent, family, friends.
- Box of irreplaceable personal valuables, like photo albums.
- Back up of computer files.
- Pyjamas, fresh sheets and towels.

After the Move:

- Be prepared to start your new position. Arrive at work early and show enthusiasm.

Hayes Specialist Recruitment offers a mnemonic for making a good first impression, IMPACT:

- *Instigate* social activities after work.
- *Manage* your time effectively.

SECTION FIVE

- *Present* yourself well.

- *Ask* questions.

- *Contribute* ideas.

- *Think* before you speak.

Explore your new city. Be a tourist at home. You can even go to the tourist information centre, ask for recommendations, and try them out. Take a city tour to get your bearings, and find out what you may want to come back to see at your leisure.

It is common for doctors to be shy and nervous about meeting new people in social situations. Our personality traits have been well described, and suggest that we feel insecure and inadequate, and like an impostor, waiting to be found out and exposed. Here are some tangible tips:

- Remember that people like to meet someone new; that they want to meet you. You are new and interesting, and they do not judge you as harshly as you do yourself.

- Remember that how you feel, your sense of uncertainly and insecurity, is not visible to others.

- Tell people that you are new, and ask them to recommend things and places for you.

- Identify and pursue your own interests—try a class or group. You will meet others with whom you already have something in common. Go for a coffee with them after.

- Decide that you are going to enjoy conversations. Start conversations.

- Ask people open-ended questions about themselves. They will like your interest and enjoy talking about themselves.

- Allow others to get to know you.

- Remember that you chose to move to this new place. Recall why you chose it, and look for these attributes consciously.

I Have What? Dealing with Chronic Illness

My resident has been recently diagnosed with a chronic medical illness. He was shocked by this. He is young and fit, and expected to be healthy for a long time. He had been experiencing some symptoms lately, but assumed they were temporary and treatable. He never expected such a serious diagnosis. He feels that his life has changed and will forever be complicated.

As doctors, we see ourselves as providing care, not requiring it. Like many of our patients, doctors also struggle to cope with chronic illness. While not generally associated with young people, chronic illnesses are actually present in 5-10% of youth. Most common are asthma and other chronic respiratory illnesses, musculoskeletal disorders, heart disease, inflammatory bowel disease, and depression.

There is little information about the prevalence of chronic mental or physical illness in physicians. Most known information is anecdotal. Despite a wide range of disabilities, it is of interest that many continue to practice medicine despite some limitations. The true prevalence among physicians may be underreported, as they tend to just accept, adapt, and carry on. Some adapt and carry on, before accepting their illness.

Doctors share some common personality traits—of being perfectionists, feeling insecure and doubting themselves, needing to be in control, wanting approval, having a strong sense of responsibility, and delaying gratification. This can impact many stages in the course of an illness—the diagnosis, treatment, and ongoing management.

The diagnosis can be delayed, because doctors delay getting help. They do not want to overreact, appear weak, or bother a colleague unnecessarily. Also, since it is "just for them", they may put it off and not make it a priority.

Treatment for physician patients can be a challenge. Often, doctors deny or minimize the problem and its symptoms, and thus do not receive adequate care. When offered treatment, doctors often like to control it themselves—managing and modifying the type of medication, dose of treatment, or self-medicating.

Effective ongoing management requires an acceptance of the chronic illness. This is not easy, as it requires grieving for the loss of one's own health, and assumptions about the future. Plans that you may have made, or assumed would be making soon, such as working up North, having a baby, or working overseas, may need to be reassessed. There can be anxiety about the outcome, understandable fears of becoming disabled, and the associated concerns about getting disability insurance or being unable to be financially independent. Reactions of fear, frustration, anger, sadness, and hopelessness are common and normal. There can be additional guilt at having added to the burden of a colleague if one's ability to work is limited.

The initial reaction of shock is entirely normal. People describe a sense of panic, waking up at night in sheer terror, a sense of dread, the daily sadness of waking up in the morning to find it has not gone away. This is natural and temporary. The first three months are always the worst. It will be easier with time.

It helps to write out your feelings, as you deal with the grief process. Doctors can all too easily intellectualize the situation, without dealing with the emotions. Writing is best done on a daily basis, putting aside about 20 minutes each day to reflect and allow your feelings. This is long enough to allow your feelings, without being so long as to feel overwhelmed by them. Doing this at night may help you sleep better and feel more rested.

Try the "I will Never" list as a strategy to identify and work through the grief, and not deny or minimize. This involves writing a header line at the top of a page such as "I will never have the healthy future I had expected." Follow this with a detailed list of things you will not have, to define the extent of the loss. This may be the most painful process you ever do, but the most effective one to define the loss and start to grieve it in a healthy manner. Do it in a safe comfortable place. Expect to cry; allow it and be gentle with yourself.

Once you are out of Denial, the next step is Anger and Protest. Again, use writing to safely and fully express your anger. The Four-Letter Technique encourages you to write out at least four letters to express your anger at your illness and people around you who can become the displaced focus of your anger. This strategy has you writing uncensored letters, without holding back, to express fully. Be careful not to leave it lying around or send it. Tear up the letter once you finish it; it has served its purpose of validating and expressing your feelings. One letter will not be enough; plan to write four. The first two or three are emotional, angry, and ugly. By the time you are at the fourth, you may be calmer and more able to understand and manage your angry feelings.

This will allow you to move on to Acceptance and Integration of this into your life. You will then find ways to accept illness and adapt to it. These stages of grieving do not follow a linear process. It is possible to complete one stage and then go back to it at a later date, although usually for a shorter period of time.

It is important to know that coping with this is a difficult process for everyone. Doctors with chronic illness are at risk of depression. Chronic medical illness has been associated with an increased prevalence of depressive symptoms. This may be due to specific biologic effects of the illness, or can be mediated by behavioural mechanisms such as limitations imposed by this illness causing gradual withdrawal from activities. It is not true that anyone would be depressed in this situation. Be alert to this possibility, and reach out to a psychiatrist or psychologist for help. Feeling depressed will greatly increase your burden, and effective treatment of this is available and will ensure an improvement in your daily functioning.

Taking care of *you* is a top priority. Pace yourself. Do not try to do all that you used to do. Even if you can do it physically, remember that this emotional process is very draining. Ask for help at work. Set more appropriate expectations and limits. Be kind to yourself, pamper yourself. Try yoga or meditation.

Reach out to family and friends. Let them take care of you and love you. Family relationships and social resources will play a key role in how you manage this emotionally. Family connectedness positively influences well-being. However, be aware that when you tell each new person, it can bring it all back as if you were reliving it again, and be painful. Expect to be drained each time. Choose whom to share this with. Be selective; you do not owe everybody this information, so just tell people who you know care about you. Let them help you. Tell more than one person, so they can share the impact of this, and there will always be someone available if you need. You can practice what you may say beforehand, since this may help you open up more easily. Don't worry about doing this perfectly. For example, there is no need or expectation to send out thank you cards immediately.

At work, it helps to inform your colleagues about your illness. Know that you did not choose this, and that you do not need to feel guilty or defensive if it causes them inconvenience. It is easier to acknowledge their help and express appreciation. Modify your working hours and workload. Be assertive of any special need you may have, such as a wheelchair or special software. Take regular breaks and holidays.

Be prepared to reassure your patients, and let them know their needs will be met by you for now, and that backup arrangements have been made, if needed.

Become educated about your illness. Don't assume that you know all you need to know because you are a doctor. Seek out web-base educational materials and resources. There may be community or on-line groups for support.

It is not easy for us as doctors to accept chronic illness or to accept care. Yet it is possible, and doing so can allow us to continue to have active and productive lives.

Aliens in the Home: Living with Adolescents

My colleague tells me that her 15-year-old daughter has become an alien. She is sullen lately, and speaks infrequently and in monosyllables. They were a close family, yet lately, she does not want to spend any time with them. She is rude, dismissive, and often critical of them. Her marks have fallen, and she does not seem to care. As doctors and parents, they have tried to encourage her to do her best, but she thinks they are nagging and wants to be making her own decisions.

Having our children go through adolescence happens to every parent. It is normal, and necessary—but it can drive us crazy. Remembering this is one of the best ways you can support them during this phase.

Adolescence is a time of transition. As adolescents, children go through a developmental stage in which they learn to separate from their parents, become individuals, and be more independent. This is normal and essential. The "terrible twos" are when children are learning to do more physically than ever before, and test their abilities, and their parents, constantly. Adolescence is a similar process, in which the new found skills are cognitive, not physical. Thus, teenagers are expanding and testing their cognitive abilities. They are learning to think differently, in a more abstract and broader manner. They can now think and reflect on things they may have never seen or experienced, such as world hunger, poverty, and peace. They try to solve these problems, and it is interesting to see them grapple enthusiastically with many of the same issues than we grappled with in our time.

As they separate and become individuals, they have their own thoughts and ideas. This can often mean doing the opposite of what they think their parents would like. It takes time to realize that whether they comply and do as expected, or defy and do the exact opposite, their behaviour is still dependent. Eventually, healthy teenagers recognize that independent thoughts can actually be the same as those of their parents.

SECTION FIVE

Separation involves a loss of the relationships and connections previously experienced with the family. Sometimes, teenagers downplay or criticize what they are losing, as a way to minimize and manage the loss. They can be moody, and unpredictable. Understanding this can help you deal more calmly with their criticism, especially when it seems to be unexpected, and unjustified.

There are times when this turbulence causes trouble at school—academically or behaviourally. It is important to keep an eye out for more serious and prolonged problems, such as depression, drug or alcohol abuse, or school failure. Talking to your teenager and suggesting follow-up with a family doctor or counsellor may be helpful.

Children of families of doctors can experience additional stress and conflicts during adolescence. Physicians may find it hard to put away their professional roles with their children. Just as they spend much of their day problem-solving and advising others on what to do, they try to do the same with their adolescent. However, since the adolescent is trying to separate, they are usually not open or interested in being advised or having their problem solved by the parent. Most physicians have high standards, are very dedicated and hard-working, and expect the same of their children. Many of them see their children as reflections of themselves, or want them to carry out their own hopes and ideals. The children struggle to set their own goals, and must deal with feelings of inadequacy if they cannot or choose to not meet their parents' goals of them. Physicians are also able to provide a privileged lifestyle for their families, and sometimes inaccurately assume that more is better. They give to their children all that they would have liked to have had, yet do not realize that this may not be what their children would like.

Healthy adolescents want to be separate, yet still want and need to be connected to the family and have rules and expectations. This is a fine balance.

I recall a two-physician family who sat in my office with their teenaged son. He was angry at them, and they were bewildered.

Here were two well-known and highly respected medical colleagues sitting in front of me, with their sullen and angry 16-year-old son, wondering where they went wrong. They both came from difficult backgrounds, and worked hard to provide a better life for their only son. They felt they had been caring, understanding, giving and flexible. They gave him all they thought he wanted; privileges and freedoms they could only have dreamed of. He had his own apartment in the basement, with a separate entrance and could come and go as he pleased, with no curfew. He had his own bank account and credit card. They had just bought him a car for his sixteenth birthday. Yet, here he was, spitting at them "You don't care about me. My friend John's parents care about him. They want him home by 10 pm, and won't go to sleep until he is safely home. You guys don't know where I am and couldn't care less if I was lying dead in a ditch all night long." Not only did he not appreciate his privileges, he did not want them and misinterpreted them as a sign of his parents not caring about him—although this could not have been further from the truth. This highlights the situation well—adolescents need rules and expectations. It is the parents' role to create rules, and the teenager's role to test them. There is no easy prescription to the healthy development of adolescents. Here are some tips that parents have passed on to me over the years.

Allow the teenager some space and a degree of separation. Respect their privacy. Give them some responsibilities. Show them that you have confidence and trust in them.

Set reasonable rules and expectations regarding behaviour. Be clear, and have specific deadlines and consequences if these are not met. Let your teenager know what the non-negotiable rules are. Include them in setting the rest of the expectations, and being a part of the decision-making process.

Teach them how to get required information, think critically, and to make good decisions for themselves. Allow them to make some poor choices and manage the consequences, but be there to support or assist them during this.

Talk openly about your concerns about sex, drugs, and alcohol. Make sure they have the information needed to make good choices. Explain how your concerns are not about restricting them or preventing them from having fun; but actually about ensuring their safety and health. Do not keep repeating this on every possible occasion, as they have heard you already.

Be open to what they want to do and be. As doctors, we want them to succeed, but may have narrow definitions of this. Recognize that they are different and unique, and may not enjoy what you do. Encourage and support them to be the best they can be, not necessarily what you think is the best.

Share your own experience as a teenager. Show them you are human, and do understand what they are going through.

Make time for them. Be available and accessible regularly. When you are with them, give them your full attention. Shopping with your teenager and bringing along a colleague to discuss medical politics is not shopping with your teenager. Driving in the car is a great place to be together and talk. It is safe, private, with no escape!

Listen actively. Ask about their thoughts and feelings. Active listening means letting them know you have heard them, but not responding with a suggestion, criticism, judgment, label, order, or lecture; or taking on their problem and solving it for them. Show respect for their thoughts and ideas.

Talk to them as you would to a friend, especially when you are angry with them. Be calm, respectful, and explain your point clearly.

Offer genuine praise. Look consciously for things they do well. Provide regular and frequent positive feedback for who they are, and what they do.

Reach out and hug them, at appropriate times and situations. They will respond positively and appreciate the intimacy. We all need reminders that we are loved.

Have fun with them. See what they are dong and are interested in, and share in it appropriately without intruding. Go to a concert, go for coffee, watch their soccer games, walk the dog together, talk about a book you have read. Laugh with them. Watch the Comedy Network, go to see a comedian, read the comics together.

Enjoy your time with them. They grow up and are gone all too soon!

It's Over: Dealing with Separation & Loss

"It's over, I'm leaving." After 23 years together, my ex-husband told me that he was not happy in our marriage and had decided to separate. Looking back on that time in my life, things seem a blur. I felt shock and disbelief. I felt rejected. I felt ashamed.

Yet, I continued to go to work each day, citing the many reasons that I couldn't take time off. There were too many patients counting on me. How would I explain it to the kids who have never seen me take a day off work; I needed to keep things as much as normal for them. In fact, I was in denial and that was my cover. I continued to do it all and go on as before–except when I was in the car driving to and from work. These became the only times in my day when I was alone, and let myself cry. Even then, I remained responsible—allowing myself to tear up at the red lights, and mopping up when the lights turned green. I think I have conditioned myself to cry at red lights for the rest of my life!

That was many years ago. I am at a different place now. Having spent a lot of my work life with the privilege of helping colleagues live healthy lives and combating the stigma of illness by speaking out about their personal experience, I decided to do the same and write this chapter to share my own personal story. I am not immune.

Being separated or divorced is to being widowed as having a mental illness is to a having a physical illness. There is an inherent sense of shame, of fault and personal responsibility, of having failed. At times, I wished there was a similar social structure of wakes and funerals for separations—that I could just put an ad in the paper letting people know it happened, giving people a place to come and give condolences and offer support, and get it all over with. Instead, I was left to tell people myself, often too tearful to be coherent. I approached work and social situations with trepidation, wondering who knew and who didn't, and who I would have to tell. I cried regularly at my local Loblaw's store, telling yet one more person I would meet there. (The manager, a good neighbor and friend, jokingly told me recently he was glad that I was feeling better; he was running out of the flowers he felt moved to give me on each such teary occasion!)

A couple of years ago, I listened intently as Dr. Michael Myers, a dear friend, colleague and mentor, gave the R.O. Jones memorial lecture at the Canadian Psychiatric Association (CPA) Annual Meeting. He spoke about "broken physicians," and the process of dealing with loss, shame, and healing. While he was speaking about colleagues with mental illness, much of it applied to my situation, too. I was still mourning the loss and feeling the shame. Michael gave me hope that there would be healing ahead.

Like many of my medical colleagues, I was no stranger to loss. We immigrated to Canada when I was four years old, leaving behind the rest of our extended family. My father was killed in a car accident when I was 11 years old. I recall the sense of panic and impending doom. I felt exactly the same when my husband told me he was leaving. I recognized the deep sense of loss encompassed the fear of loss of my other extended family, especially my father-in-law, with whom I am very close.

The sense of shame ran deep. I was "found out"—a fraud. I "pretended" to help my colleagues improve their relationships and live better lives; I failed at doing this myself. For months, I could not look people in the eye. I asked myself what more I could have done. I found it hard to tell people my husband and I were no longer together, bracing myself for the expected (but never received) lecture on how it was my fault, that I should have tried harder, done more.

My initial response was to do what most highly functioning people do when we are feeling stress—do more. I worked harder than ever, seeing patients, assuming the OPA presidency, writing, doing more talks. It was far easier to be out of town presenting than to be alone in the house on a weekend when the boys were not with me.

I soon realized that I was surrounded by fantastic people who cared about me—me as a person, and not me as part of a couple. My family was amazingly supportive. The beauty of having my mother and so many sisters close by is that they always ensured one of them was around to be with me—a call schedule of sorts! My friends were all there, telling me I was a good person and would get through this. My psychiatry journal club members surrounded me with care and support. One of my dearest friends from medical school encouraged me to ask myself each day "What's good about this?" Some days, it was almost impossible to answer that, but having asked it, I always found an answer.

One of my sons asked, "How many doctors does it take to help the Doctors' Doctor?"

I replied, "At last count, I think it's 42."

"Isn't that the Meaning of Life, Mom?"

Slowly, the healing started. As I reached out to family and friends, I learned how to let others take care of me. I started to believe the good things they told me about myself and my strengths. I took time to let myself feel, cry, and let go. I spent one New Year's holiday purposely alone, enjoying not one, but two, pyjama days! I focused on self care routines—sleeping better, regular exercise, nutrition. I took salsa dance classes, cooking workshops, and yoga lessons. Serenity arose from confusion. I learned to acknowledge and let go of the shame and guilt. There was a resulting greater sense of control, confidence, hope, and dignity. The fog lifted.

My sons have been so wonderful. We have had some memorable holidays, discovering new continents together. They are full of humor, and every day we laugh together, a good reminder of what did not change. They are wonderful, supportive, and loving, and I am a proud and happy mother.

About three years later, my oldest son was off to university. The three boys sat me down before he left. The twins told me that they, too, would be heading off the following year, and did not want to worry about me. They encouraged me to start dating. "We know you are happy on your own, but it would be great if you met someone. We have already told our friends' parents to look for someone for you." They were very supportive, and ready to accept anyone…with one condition "He has to adore you." A chance meeting with a colleague occurred a few months later, which led to our marriage last year. He is a very special person, kind, gentle, and loving (and yes, he adores me).

A close friend, colleague, and author of the self-help book, *On Your Own Again*, Keith Anderson, chronicles the progress of dealing with separation and loss. It is reassuring to know that this is a process, and things do improve, and one can re-establish a balance in life again. Some people prefer to remain on their own and enjoy newfound independence, some actively seek a new relationship, and others, like me, do neither but remain open and recognize someone special when they meet them. Regardless, there is hope that one can build a new life and move forward.

SECTION FIVE

The Kids Are Driving...Me Crazy

Life changed for me again last week. The 16-year old twins passed their G2 driving exam. I now have two new drivers in the house...and a lot of mixed feelings.

They had been working hard for this and I was happy for them. They went directly to the Ministry of Transport on their sixteenth birthday, to write the initial exam. Everywhere we had gone in the past eight months, I had let them drive, (one on the way there, the other on the way back), and so had lots of time to know they were both good, careful drivers. They had taken the driver's training course and passed it successfully. And, I had been waiting for them to drive themselves to many of the various lessons, practices, and rehearsals. So, why was I feeling so uncertain? It was a big step, with a lot of freedom, independence and responsibility. Were they ready for this? More importantly, was I?

The first test came immediately. The very next day after they got their G2 licenses, they had planned to drive to school, and then go downtown to meet their friends to skate on the canal and check out the sculptures during the Winterlude Festival, and then go for dinner afterwards. However, Ottawa was bracing for a 30 cm snowstorm. I listened to the radio weather report that morning, and my first instinct was to tell them they could not drive as planned. Luckily, they were still asleep! I got the chance to think about it further, and realized this was only one of many solutions. In fact, if they were going to learn to drive in bad weather, it may as well be in the same city as me, when I could be available to them.

As doctors, we are used to making decisions for others. We gather data and come to a conclusion. We sometimes forget that this is only possible because our patients allow us to do so. The other people in our lives do not always give us that same control. Adolescents are especially interested in keeping such control and making their own decisions; in fact, the developmental task at this stage of life is Separation and Individuation. Their job is to learn to separate healthily from their parents and make their own choices as an individual; our task as parents is to help them learn how to do so. Since they were born, my decisions for them and limits that I set were all focused on ensuring their health and safety. I took the opportunity to share my concerns with them about their health and safety in this particular situation, and then explore together necessary preparations and precautions. We spoke about how to make sure they had warm clothing, blankets and food in the car, a shovel in case they got stuck in an unplowed street, a full gas tank, a cell phone (that was turned on), and a CAA card that they had learned how to use.

They listened carefully and headed off. I kept busy and filled my day, until I finally heard the garage door go up, the car doors close in the garage, and their happy voices in the mudroom. I heard about how they did need the shovel, having got stuck on their way home, in our own street a few feet from the end of driveway. I was proud of them, their new skills, and their confidence. I was excited about the freedom I could envision for me ahead.

I drove to work that morning on my own, for the first time, not needing to drive the boys to school on the way. I started to talk, then realized they were not there to listen. I had not realized how I had become used to that time together, and thought about how wonderful it had been to drive them places. That was probably when we had had our best conversations, since they were often alone with me, held hostage and stuck in the seat beside me, but without direct eye contact, and knew the discussion was time-limited and would not go on forever. I should have appreciated every one of those minutes more, instead of wishing some of them away. We are in a new phase again, an exciting new start full of freedoms and promise for all of us.

SECTION FIVE

New Beginnings: Moving House

"It's the Year of the Rat," she said. "New beginnings. It's the start of a 12 year cycle in the Chinese calendar." This year is supposed to be a year of plenty, bringing opportunity, and good prospects. We are sitting at the kitchen table in my new house, my friend and I, having a drink and celebrating my new beginning. I have just moved, and the boxes are barely opened and put away. It is nice to see walls and floor, instead of boxes and piles of furniture.

I reflected on what she had said. All day and all around me, I watch people dealing with change and transitions. Life brings such change—people get married, widowed, separated, or divorced; people have new babies, send their kids off to school and then to university; people have serious illnesses; people get hired, fired, or promoted at work; people move, rent, buy, and sell houses.

Each situation is a new beginning, after the end of something else.

In his book, *Transitions: Making Sense of Life's Changes*, William Bridges describes the three phases of a transition. There is an End, followed by a period of Confusion and Distress, and then a New Beginning. Regardless of what the change is, all of us go through these stages. Dealing with the end of something requires us to go through the process of grief, with a sense of loss and regret, and possibly shame and confusion. While it may be a bit easier if we have chosen the change, as I did with this house move, the choice does not entitle us to avoid the grief process. Ultimately, we have to let go of the old way, so we can move on and embrace the new beginning.

My recent move asks me to do the same—to let go and move on. I have just moved out of a house in which I lived for about 20 years, and decided that this would be a good opportunity to downsize, simplify, and clear out clutter. I had seriously under-estimated how much effort this would take...or perhaps I did know and so was putting it off. As a result, I left the bulk of the sorting and packing to the last month. This proved to be a huge task. As I touched everything in the house, considering whether it would have a place in the new house, I realized that everything had a history and memory attached, and that dealing with this would add to the energy that this task would take. There were old toys, outgrown and outdated clothes, magazines and cards and letters, photographs, school art and creative writing projects, books, VHS movies, dishes...Luckily, my sisters and friends helped me to be first sentimental, and then brutal. I was allowed to have the memory one last time, and then put the item in the give-away pile. The children were doing the same. I came across one of them with tears in his eyes as he, just home after his first year of university, looked at a photograph of himself on the first day of kindergarten. Later, the twins laughed uproariously at a story they had made up in Grade 2 about Godzilla and alien invaders, complete with hand drawn pictures. We were all happy to know that our pile of things that we had decided not to take with us would be going to immigrant and women's shelters, and that others would benefit from them.

The new house is great. Our things fit there perfectly, and we no longer remember much of what we have let go. We have a few new things that fit better here. The appliances are finally in; the furniture is in place, the pictures are hung up on the walls. The cable, phone, and internet are finally hooked up; and the 27 calls it took us to achieve that will soon be forgotten. It feels like we have been here much longer than the past week. Our friends visit us here now, even those from our old neighborhood. This morning, I drove to work along the new route, almost absent-mindedly. A nice young couple, recently graduated from medical school and starting their residencies, will move in to our old home and start the next phase of their lives—the same stage that we were in when we first moved there. Already we have let go and are moving on.

SECTION FIVE

As The Nest Empties

Thanksgiving weekend is over, and I find myself sending my son back to university with pride mingled with sadness after his first visit home. I know that I am in good company; most of our friends and colleagues with children of similar age are all at this stage. I recall when we spoke about finishing med school or residencies so we could start a family. Now the kids are moving away. How did we get here so fast?

I recall the boys as babies, staying awake nights with them, helping them settle back to sleep while sacrificing my own sleep; and dreaming of where else I could be and what else I could be doing. A weekend, actually a day, or even just an hour to myself would have been welcomed. I distinctly recall my pleasure in finally having the time to finish a cup of tea—even that had been a rare treat for several years. Going to the office was a break—I could actually eat lunch in peace, or go to the bathroom by myself! I recall laughing with an older colleague who told me to enjoy this, as the "Empty Nest Syndrome" was tough for him and his wife. Yeah sure, I thought; I'd miss the kids...sure, I'd miss the long nights with the kids waking up with wet diapers, or lost soothers, or for no apparent reason; or the twins graciously offering their colic in stereo.

Over the years, I continued the dreams of having time to myself—no last minute homework projects that had me rushing out for poster board at 8:55 p.m.; no complaints about dirty dishes or socks in the family room or towels on the floor; no soccer practices or music lessons to drive to; no phone calls that were never answered by the kids but were never for me.

Then, this past January, my eldest son applied to university. I was proud and excited for him, and tried to help in whatever small way I could. I listened to him debating one program over another, listened as he read aloud the drafts of his personal statements, where he tried to express his interest and desire for the programs, and helped him prepare for interviews in other cities, and drove him there and back. In April, he heard he was accepted to his top choice in Toronto, and the planning began. I started to keep a list of all that he would need, (I am happy to share this 97 item list and have it available to any of you as a Word document!) and spent the summer off and on acquiring these items when I was able to leave the office early. That these things all fit into a van, and into his dorm room, remains a miracle. I left him there, sorting out the details of his classes schedule, the text book list, the meal plan, and Frosh Week. Looking back, I kept too busy to be sentimental or to be aware of how much I would miss him.

In fact, I can now see that he has been thoughtfully preparing me for this for a few years. In high school, he began to make new friends whose parents I had never met, went out on weekends, started to drive, got a bank debit card, and was becoming more independent and taking on more responsibility. At the end of the summer, he taught me how to text and use Skype so we could connect regularly albeit briefly while he was away. Interestingly, it seems that just as things were starting to get better; it was time for him to go. Yet, he was able to show me all he had learned and reassure me that he would be fine. He is managing his new routine and responsibilities, doing it his way, communicating and staying connected, but leaving me to trust his opinions and decisions.

The Empty Nest Syndrome is not an actual psychiatric diagnosis. It refers to the general feeling of loneliness that a parent or guardian feels when one or more children leave the home, no longer live with them, or need day-to-day care. It is most common in the fall when children leave for university, or when children get married. It is natural, normal, even necessary, for a parent to feel a sense of sadness. A colleague of mine once told me what his mother said to him. "The day the last one of you kids left the house was the happiest day of my life...The next day was the saddest."

More troubling reactions can occur, however. If a parent feels extreme sadness or loneliness, feels that their useful life has ended, cries excessively, or no longer wants to go out or go to work—and this lasts longer than a week or two, professional help is indicated. The departure has likely tapped into other issues of loss and precipitated depression.

I have found some tips to help me in this transition. Some I have come across on my own, some are offered by friends who stumbled upon them. I am happy to pass them on.

Remember that we have successfully managed many other transitions in the past—university, med school, residency, setting up practice. We can do this one, too.

Keep in mind that your child is taking an important step in their life; this is not about us. Your child is working through the process of Separation and Individuation, a normal and necessary process of child development, as described by Margaret Mahler, which allows the child to separate from the parents and successfully gain a sense of individual identity. Erik Erikson, a noted psychoanalyst, similarly described eight stages of development that we all go through in life. Each is related to a specific development task or issue, and the achievement of each task allows us to healthily succeed and proceed to the next stage. Adolescence is Erikson's fifth stage, between 12 and 18 years of age, and the basic conflict to be resolved here is Identity vs. Role Confusion. Social relationships and experiences during this stage allow the teen to develop a healthy sense of self and identity. Failure to do so results in identity and role confusion.

Here are a few strategies shared by parents which can help you manage this phase successfully.

Ration your phone calls to once or twice a week. It is okay if they call you more often. Try to set aside a regular time to call, so you can both fit it into your schedules.

Try to text or email them; it is easier for them to reply on their own time, and it may be easier to communicate feelings with less emotions. Funny, light notes about what is going on at home work well.

If they are not happy there, try not to be too happy. Encourage them to keep trying, reassure them, and support them to continue.

If they need something, try to walk them through how to do/get it, not do it for them. We are there to support them, not to smother them.

Talk to your friends, especially those who have gone or are going through a similar process. They are a huge source of support and advice.

Ask yourself "What's good about this?" and plan to take advantage of that benefit. For example, use the time gained from not having to drive them places to start your regular exercise program, or enjoy the extra bedroom to invite out-of-town friends to visit.

Identify things that you have always wanted to do, and start now. This is a great time for new activities or interests, outside medicine.

Do not stay at work longer, just because you may not have kids at home that need you to come home. Leave the office or hospital as before, and find new, fun things to do without kids.

While I do miss my son, and know that it is never easy to let go, I know it is the right thing to do and that he is ready for it. The journey from cradle to college has been complicated, perplexing, fulfilling, and satisfying. I remember an email he sent to me after a couple of weeks of classes. "I love it here. I feel that I am in exactly the right place for this stage in my life." What a wonderful thing for a parent to hear! I look forward to the next stage in this journey, where I get to enjoy my relationship with the amazing young adult he has become.

SECTION FIVE

Achieving Successful Retirement

"Okay, it's now the New Year. Let's get on with it," my patient said grudgingly, as if we were about to start on a root canal procedure. I realized he was speaking about the discussion of his retirement plans, a topic he had been deferring for several months now. He just could not bring himself to consider retiring from medicine, after being a doctor for over four decades.

This was such a far cry from the myth of "Freedom 55"! What a great sell that was; the ideal of the perfect retirement. The ads showed pictures of gorgeous sandy beaches and palm trees; lounging chairs and hot tubs and hammocks; drinks with umbrellas; and older couples youthfully laughing, playing, and walking on the beach at sunset. It depicted work as "not fun," and retirement as "fun." There was a clear distinction, with three separate phases:

1. Full time work.
2. The gold watch.
3. Full time leisure.

There was a clear goal, to get from Phase 1 to 3 as early as possible.

Yet, this has changed with a changing world. People are living longer, are healthier when older, and need to finance more years of life. People are better educated, and want to continue to do something as they get older. As within medicine, people often got their sense of power from their workplace and want to maintain this. Our work defines us, and we also want to maintain this sense of self.

Mandatory retirement is mostly gone. In 1990, a Canadian legal case, McKinney vs. University of Guelph, was decided in favor of the employer, stating that forced retirement at age 65 was within reasonable limits under section 1 of the Canadian Charter of Human Rights. This is now being questioned, as it is increasingly considered to be discriminatory under section 15 of the Charter. Forcing employees to retire has become a human rights issue. Manitoba, Quebec, Alberta, and PEI all have legislation to protect employees from age discrimination after age 65 years. On December 12, 2006, Ontario amended its Human Rights code to give employees the same protection and end mandatory retirement.

Sir William Osler, known as the Father of Modern Medicine, gave a famous and controversial speech upon his appointment to Oxford as their Regis Professor of Medicine, in 1905 (at age 56 years himself). He stated that "the effective, moving, vitalizing work of the world is done between the ages of twenty-five and forty," and that "a person over 50 has little to contribute to society and stands in the way of progress." The changing world requires a change in attitude. "Old" used to be a negative concept, associated with a sense of being less productive and less efficient. In reality, as one ages, many abilities are unchanged. If one's capacity decreases, it is compensated by increased experience. New attitudes must make our older colleagues feel welcome and respected in the workplace, especially as they are needed in the face of serious work shortages.

A 2005 HSBC Survey showed that only 22% of Canadians see retirement as pure rest and relaxation. Most of us see this phase as a time for reinvention, pursuing lost ambitions, or taking on new personal challenges. The Harris County Medical Society Study showed that most physicians are pleased with retirement, with 33% stating that these were the happiest years. Understandably, the first year of retirement was felt to be the most stressful. Most are financially comfortable. The healthiest ones were the ones who were the best emotionally prepared.

The single best way to prepare for a healthy retirement is to start early—at least by the age of 45 years. Basically, we will need to replace 40-60 (or more!) hours of work with other meaningful activities. It is hard to find new interests overnight. We need to identify these early, and start to practice, and see if we will actually enjoy them. This process of transition takes about two full years, and involves anticipating and accommodating physical and emotional changes, and grieving the inherent losses.

SECTION FIVE

There are emotional challenges. The end of a long and successful medical career leads to multiple changes and can bring about an acute sense of loss. There can be a loss of self-worth, of our own identity as a physician. Now, who are we and what is our role in society? Suddenly, there is no place to go, no familiar structure and routine to our days, and a sense of isolation as much of our social life was centered on our work.

There are professional challenges. It can be difficult to slow down, with a lack of support for coverage or availability of locums. Some medical groups require colleagues to take full call, even if they are cutting back hours at work. Professional organizations still require payment of full professional fees, regardless of how much one works. As we work less, we can feel excluded and alone, and miss colleagues and the networking within medicine.

There are financial challenges. How much is enough to retire? We need to feel that we have enough money to do all the things we want to do, now that we have more time to do them. Regular consultations with financial advisors will greatly assist in the planning and creation of the savings required. Again, we need to start early to plan for this, and set realistic and flexible goals.

Work in later years is now actually a blend of retirement and work. This can include working part-time; mentoring junior colleagues and sharing skills and knowledge; remodelling job skills into volunteer work, or self employment. In medicine, there are many options. One can offer to do locums for younger colleagues for sabbaticals, maternity leaves, study leaves, and holidays; or do locums in under-serviced areas such as the Canadian North. One can sign up for short term missions or disaster relief programs. We can teach in a developing nation. We can modify our regular work, such as run a specialized clinic or assist a colleague. We can serve on review committees and boards. We can edit, review, and write. We can teach, or focus on research we did not make time to do earlier in our career.

Here are some key steps in planning for retirement:

- Start planning early. It is never too early to think about it.

- Talk to other retirees about what worked and what did not work.

- Talk to those you live with. It is *our*, not *my*, retirement.

- Invest in your relationship now, because you will be spending more time together. Appreciate, praise, and apologize if needed.

- Determine how connected you want to be to your old work place. This will help in deciding what you will want to do and where.

- Identify interests and start to practice what you think you want to do once you retire. Finding meaningful activities may take a year or more.

- Stop before you start. Even if you want to do something else, first take a few months and do nothing. "Do nothing until you can't stand it anymore." You will then likely want to be busy again.

- Do the things you want to do in life while you still can. Don't put it off until later. Later is now.

- Help patients plan for transition. Discourage dependency, notify them about two to three months in advance, transfer charts or tell how to access them, and announce it in the paper.

- Consider your colleagues. Express appreciation, and plan to stay connected.

Ken Spencer, former CEO of Creo Products, summed it up well when he said, "Retirement is not about doing nothing. It is about doing what you want to do, with the people you want to do it with."

Closing Your Practice

For someone who does not like change and treasures stability and security, I have sure experienced more than my share of it in recent years. So, who would have thought that I would actually choose to make another huge change to my life? Yet, that's exactly what I did. At the end of August, after almost twenty years, I closed my office practice.

It was a huge leap for me. Yet, it seemed the time was right. A long office lease was ending, and the twins were going off to university and were more independent. If I were ever going to make a change, this was the time.

I had been thinking about doing something different for a while. Initially, these thoughts would be fleeting, but regular. I had trained as a child psychiatrist, yet by serendipity found myself with a few colleagues as patients, which led to the privilege and honor of exclusively treating physicians in my private practice for most of twenty years. Over the years, I watched the area of physician health expand until there is now a good network of resources available. Recently, there were times when I felt like I did as a child psychiatrist, when I would treat a beautiful, anxious seven-year-old girl, only to have to send her back into the dysfunctional family that helped to create and perpetuate the anxiety. I questioned what I would have done as a child psychiatrist. There would need to be additional family therapy, and education for parenting skills. It made me think about how I could do translate this within the medical workplace "family". I could focus on educating the leaders on how to create healthy medical workplaces, and on working with medical teams on improving their sense of engagement, connection, collegiality, and communication skills. Recently, a colleague contacted me to tell me he was taking over the role as Chair of a large department, and knew that I had helped his predecessor. He asked me, "Do I have to wait until I feel overwhelmed and get depressed, or can I come see you now?" In fact, as a psychiatrist, I really did need him to have the diagnosis first; but this got me thinking again.

STRENGTH TRAINING AFTER INJURY

I am embarking on the next phase of my career, still focusing on Physician Health, but now from the perspective of Primary Prevention to expand the spectrum. I have taken courses and workshops and got my certificate in Coaching, so I work with physician executives. This is exciting; yet scary, especially the business and financial part. It is not covered by OHIP, the provincial health plan, so I have to set up a real business, and learn to market and promote myself as a consultant and coach. At times, I wonder "What am I doing? I have three sons in university—absolutely the wrong time to give up a stable income!" Yet, I balance that with my new goals, reminding myself that physician health needs to envelop a proactive approach address workplace issues, too; and that I have the experience, knowledge, and training to succeed.

Closing up a practice is amazingly difficult. I truly underestimated the energy it would take. I started to tell my patients six months in advance, and both me and my patients grieved the associated loss, although much of mine was necessarily and appropriately private. We went through Denial; "You can't do that" or "I dreamed that you had change your mind; is that true?" Anger; "How can you abandon me?" Protest; "It's not fair; we were doing so well." Bargaining; "Perhaps you can still fit me in once a month?" Sadness; "I am really going to miss you. " And, finally, Acceptance; "Thank you for all you have done. You have really helped me, and I know you will do more as you reach a broader audience."

In my office, I listened, validated feelings, accepted all the various reactions and gave permission for them to be expressed and understood and addressed. Yet, I was exhausted at the end of each afternoon. For months, I would go home and fall asleep before dinner; I had not done that since I was expecting the twins. I started to be unable to multitask, was misplacing things, and would not even finish sentences. I realized how drained I was, and made time for people and activities that would help me to reenergize. I asked myself "What's good about this?" reminding myself why I was making the change, what I had hoped to achieve. I told myself it would be better as I could now have more collegial relationships with colleagues. Treating colleagues was very rewarding, but had been very isolating. Every time someone came to see me in the office, I would lose another colleague or friend, as new roles and rules came into play. That did not need to keep happening any more.

As the final weeks approached, the patients were primarily happy and excited for me, offering congratulations, support, and thanks. I don't think I am alone in this; receiving kindness and care from others is my undoing. My eyes refused to stay dry as colleagues in my office shed their own tears as they spoke beautifully touching words of gratitude, extended hugs, brought thoughtful gifts for me to enjoy with my family, made donations to the United Way on my behalf, offered to be available to help my sons who were attending university in their cities, and even offered to help me pack my office.

I had patients booked until the end of the last afternoon. Then, I closed the door, closed my appointment book, and pulled up a box to pack.

It is now weeks later. My days have a new and different rhythm and structure. My new business is established and incorporated, has a name and a logo, and is off to a great start. I am amazed by how well things have progressed, and how I do not have to do much to convince people of what I can offer them now. It is exciting to broaden the spectrum of physician health and move beyond the individual treatment focus and approach; to help in making systemic changes to maintain and sustain the health of physicians.

SECTION SIX

PERFORMANCE ENHANCEMENT: MANAGING YOUR CAREER IN MEDICINE

•

Why Attend Medical Conferences? Why Not!

It's medical conference season. I find myself travelling away from home more in the fall to present and attend conferences. Yet another flight; yet another hotel. Good thing I really love going to conferences. I love learning new things, meeting new people, seeing new places. As I reflect more on this, I realize that there are four main reasons that we doctors attend medical conferences—to learn, network, travel, and relax—and while there needs to be one of these reasons present, any combination of the four are possible.

We go to conferences to learn. This is still one of the best ways to maintain and update our education, knowledge and skills. It's like one-stop shopping for the science and art of medicine. We learn a great amount in one location, from a number of experts, on a variety of related topics. While much of our continuing education is now available on line, attending in person remains the best way to hone a specific skill set.

We go to conferences to network, to meet our colleagues and friends and get caught up. Professional connections are made and developed. We meet speakers, top researchers, and clinicians who share our area of interest, and can also share experience and expertise, and make plans to collaborate in the future. Personal connections are made, too. There is the regular group of people one meets every year at the same conference. Little traditions and rituals can develop. I have a group of women colleagues that plan to go to the same conference, and manage an annual day at the spa together while we are there. Then there is the group that attends another conference together and has the "martini moment" the first evening there. However, it's not just a place to meet peers from other cities. I am embarrassed to say that there are some colleagues from my home town that I only see in other cities at conferences. We just seem to get too busy to socialize at home.

Meeting peers at conferences can sometimes be an emotionally difficult experience, however. It can bring out feelings of competition, insecurity, or a sense of failure. There are times when we listen to what others are doing and how much they have achieved, and feel our own achievements pale in comparison. "He was a classmate of mine, and while I just see patients in the office, he has gone on to develop an international reputation and be the world expert in this field." We can feel intimidated, feel too shy to speak up, say hello, or ask (we think, stupid) questions. It helps to remember that we have all achieved a great deal, just by getting into and completing medical school—99% of the people in the world do not do this. We all make choices; we have made ours to practice medicine the way we do and our colleagues have made theirs. There is no right choice; they are different and complementary, and there is a role and need for us all. A good goal when we go to a conference is to *meet two new people*, to consciously push past our personal insecurities and reach out and talk to two people we do not know. While hard to start, it yields amazing results!

We go to conferences to travel. It is a great way to go to a new city or country, and explore the area in between sessions. Many of us extend the trip at either end, planning an extra day or two to tour the location. The extra time it may take to plan and prepare for this pays off when we sample local sounds, sights, and tastes. Many conferences plan special tours and outings for conference delegates and their families, and it is definitely worth taking advantage of these as they have been well planned by the host city. The highlight of a recent conference in Edinburgh was a private dinner at Edinburgh Castle, complete with our own tour of the crown jewels, being piped in to dinner, the ceremonial serving of the haggis, Scotch tasting, and a full Highland band leading the procession at the end of a memorable evening.

We go to conferences to relax; "A change is as good as a rest." While we are still working and learning, our usual daily responsibilities of work are left behind—we do not have to see patients, run an office, or teach, and can just focus on our own learning needs. Colleagues agree that it is much harder to attend a conference in their own city, as they usually try to do it all, be available, and find themselves running around and not able to relax as easily. Even if one is presenting at a conference, the rest of the day is available for one's own interests, without our usual work responsibilities. Even if our families join us, we are more able to spend quality or fun time with them, doing new things without the usual concerns about cooking, cleaning, and driving to evening lessons, practices, and rehearsals.

A reminder is in order—while we are making new friends and acquaintances, it helps to remember that this is still a professional endeavour, and our behaviour needs to be in keeping with this. So, while it is great to socialize, to go out for a drink, (even sing karaoke in Scottish pubs!), we need to remain in control so we can best enjoy ourselves, our colleagues, and the situation.

Finally, as conferences are positive for us in so many ways, use the Tarzan Rule to keep them happening. While swinging through the jungle, Tarzan does not let go of one vine without having the next one in hand. Do not leave a conference without having planned your next one!

PERFORMANCE ENHANCEMENT

Have a Mentor: Be a Mentor

It has been said that mentoring is the most important tool in becoming the professional that we want to be. I shall always remember with gratitude the key people who have been instrumental to my career. They were there at the right time, guiding me, supporting me, and encouraging me to do more than I would have attempted on my own. I am part of a unique journal club. While all of us are psychiatrists, all of us in the group also shared the same amazing mentor, who brought us together during our training, believed in us, and taught us how to balance excellence in medicine and excellence as a human being. Our success is a testament to him and his mentoring.

What is a mentor? A mentor is a teacher, guide, coach, supporter, promoter, advisor, counsellor, promoter, sponsor, and nurturer. Usually, it is someone who has been there—wherever it is that you want to go. It must be someone you can trust, who wants to help you succeed, and who will be gratified by your success.

The process of mentorship involves two people with a common interest, differing levels of experience and seniority, working together, with a common goal to further the interests of the most junior person.

From your mentor, you can hope to gain advice and experience. Your mentor can help you develop a supportive work environment, become more visible, and give you a sense of belonging. they are able to advocate for you and act as a role model.

Why would someone devote such time and effort to be a mentor to you? They gain recognition and the respect of their peers. Most mentors describe a sense of personal satisfaction, and truly enjoy the gratification of enhancing someone else's development.

Mentors are useful at the beginning of your career, at a turning point in your professional life, or when you have a special role or expectation. For example, a mentor can teach you how to set up your own practice, and negotiate a lease. If you later decide that you want to do more research, a mentor who is currently doing research would be invaluable. If you want to start writing and publishing, find someone who is doing just that. You can turn to a mentor for advice on how to balance a career and young children, find a nanny, and not feel too guilty when you head out each morning. When you are applying for university promotion, a mentor can help you put your package together, present your experiences in the best possible way, and help you reach your goal.

There are no real rules for obtaining a mentor. There are several formal peer mentoring programs—at academic institutions; in medical schools and residency programs; within hospital departments; in local, provincial, and national specialty and medical societies. Explore these, as they are well organized, and supported by eager, experienced, supportive colleagues. Mentors are also available informally. Often, finding a great mentor is pure luck! It helps if you can plan, assess, and identify your needs. Review names of colleagues who could be of potential help to you. The best advice I can offer is to look around, find someone who is doing what you would like to do (and seems happy doing it!), and reach out to them. Don't be shy; approach them. Although they may seem too busy and are not openly offering their availability as a mentor, they are usually flattered and pleased to do so when approached. There is no perfect mentor. It can be a peer or a supervisor, and can be from within or outside of medicine. Remember, this is not a marriage, and you do not have to be monogamous. You can have more than one mentor at a time!

Don't worry about "repaying" your mentor. This is not expected or wanted. The best thing you can do is to learn the most from what they can give to you. It is like a temporary loan—pass it on to someone else at a later point.

Don't forget that even while you are seeking some help, there is still much you can offer to another junior colleague at the same time. You could use a mentor. You could be a mentor.

PERFORMANCE ENHANCEMENT

Having a mentor is the most important factor in becoming the professional you want to be.

SECTION SIX

Mentorship: Become the Professional You Want to Be

At a recent Journal Club, I looked around at the ten of us who have been meeting monthly since we finished our residency about twenty years ago. One of the things that we share in common is being mentored as residents by the same person. He was an amazing senior colleague. As the Chief of the department, he was very busy, yet he always made time for us. He let us take responsibility, always supported decisions we made, took us for coffee daily, and taught us the both the art and the science of medicine. It is largely due to his influence that each of our group chose to become psychiatrists.

In recent years, we have seen an increase in formal mentorship programs in medicine, such as within medical schools, residency programs, specialty organizations, groups of researchers, and for women physicians. These have been well received, and are known to serve the profession well. Mentoring is not a new management technique. Humans have always learned by example and apprenticeship and coaching. This can occur in any organization—both formally and informally.

It is obvious that the mentees have much to gain from such a relationship. It has been said that mentoring is the most important tool in becoming the professional we want to be. In mentoring, an older, wiser, more experienced person assists another to learn and grow. The mentor acts as a teacher, guide, coach, sponsor, advisor, counsellor, supporter, promoter, nurturer, and protector. The mentor is someone who has been there, can be trusted, and is genuinely gratified by the success of another.

Yet, what's in it for the mentor? Many of us may want to become mentors, but balk at the amount of time and energy it may involve. It is an extra undertaking—on top of the huge job we already have. The roles are not always clear. If there is no extra money, no protected time for this, yet we are asked to assume more responsibility, why would we want to do it?

While the goal of mentorship is usually focused on promoting the growth and interest of the person being mentored, it would be a mistake to assume that the mentor gains nothing from this process. Research in the mentoring literature clearly demonstrates these gains. Having served as a mentor, both informally and formally, for medical students, residents in psychiatry, and junior colleagues, I can personally attest to this.

Career enhancement; The career of the mentor is boosted by these activities. Mentors receive increased visibility and recognition from their peers. Those who develop a reputation as being helpers in any organization generally enjoy higher status within the system. This shows a commitment to the profession. There may be greater opportunities for grants or research awards, if the mentee is interested in joining in this work. Being a mentor allows one to develop and enhance ones own personal style of leadership. I have been invited to speak at many conferences or workshops by colleagues who I had previously mentored in their training. It is so touching to have such personal introductions and realize that I have made a difference to them and they have remembered it after all these years.

Building networks; A mentor can develop a close relationship with the mentee that may help them in the future. A sense of loyalty is fostered. New support networks with other professionals can result, promoting collegiality. As a mentor, one can more easily spot talent for later recruitment. Every year that I served as a mentor to the medical students, I was thrilled when one of them decided to choose psychiatry as a speciality. It feels great to know that I had been able to be a positive role model, transfer my enthusiasm, and make psychiatry an appealing option for them.

Increased personal learning; Being a mentor offers an opportunity for increased personal growth and self-awareness, and the chance to review and reflect on what one has attained and achieved as you pass it on to another. One can learn new perspectives and approaches, and feel a sense of rejuvenation, as links are gained to younger, less experienced colleagues. Mentorship enables the enhancement of communication skills, such as coaching, listening, and counselling. I always learn something from the mentees. They are keen and eager to learn and experience all they can. They have such an innocent and infectious excitement for medicine, and constantly remind me of why I chose to be a doctor in the first place. I recapture the magic and the meaning of medicine.

Increased sense of satisfaction; There is great emotional pleasure as we watch another person grow and mature, and help motivate them to achieve their full potential and succeed. It leads to a sense of being needed and recognized professionally, while engaging in a meaningful volunteer activity. Some of the medical students in my mentor group have asked me to give them their diploma when they graduate. This is heady stuff. I feel so honoured to have been a part of their education, and am truly filled with pride and joy at their achievements.

"Why did you do all this for me?" [Wilbur] asked. "I don't deserve it. I've never done anything for you."

"You have been my friend," replied Charlotte…"By helping you, perhaps I was trying to lift my life a trifle. Heaven knows, anyone's life can stand a little of that."

—— E. B. White, *Charlotte's Web*

I Thought it would Suck, but it Didn't

I cross my fingers as I pick up the phone to make the call. This is the fifth call I have made this evening for this purpose, and I hope that I am on a winning streak. As Past-President of the Ontario Psychiatric Association, it is my duty to head the Nominations process and ensure that we have a full slate of offices for the coming year's OPA Council. Easier said than done! I am sure that this is a sign of the stressful times that we now live and work in. Everyone seems too busy; it is not easy to get colleagues to come out to yet another event, and donate their time to yet another organization.

This is not specific to the OPA. In fact, other than to the Ontario Medical Association, to which all physicians in Ontario must belong, according to the Rand Formula, numerous other medical associations are dealing with the same issue. Membership numbers are declining, and up to 25% of the current membership will be retiring in the coming decade. Even among groups where the membership rate is high and show support by a financial contribution, the members are not actually playing an active role in the workings of the organization. Annual meetings are being scaled down, annual dinners are being modified or cancelled, and regular get-togethers are being deferred as fewer physicians take time to attend.

This is also not specific to medical organizations. I have heard similar laments in the academic arena, where many committees are having trouble recruiting new members. Other professions, such as law, dentistry, and business, also share this concern. People are just not coming out to events after work.

A similar pattern is seen throughout our western culture, as described by Professor Robert Putnam from Harvard in his 1995 essay, *Bowling Alone: America's Declining Social Capital*. About 25% fewer voters are turning out at US national elections. A Roper survey showed that the number of Americans who attend public meetings has fallen since 1973 by about a third. There are similar declines in the numbers of people attending political speeches and rallies, serving on committees of local organizations, belonging to church-related groups, or having memberships in labor unions. The numbers of volunteers for civic organizations, such as Boy Scouts and Red Cross have declined markedly, by as much as 60% since 1970. Fraternal organizations such as the Lions, Shriners, Jaycees and the Masons have also witnessed substantial drops in memberships.

Interestingly, just today, I listened to a morning radio program on my way to work. Representatives from two community organizations in Ottawa were being interviewed. One was an active urban young neighborhood, which had lots of events and activities, and lots of volunteers, "often more than we need." The other one was a suburban older neighborhood where the children were mostly grown up and headed off to university, and the parents were quieter and less involved. The latter group was appealing to the community to come out and join the association, but acknowledged that there seemed to be little impetus to do so. The discussion centred on the adage that "Bad news is good news" to groups, and that people need to feel a sense of being threatened or have to deal with unwanted change to become actively involved. It is clear that a sense of ownership is required for involvement, that is, "What's In It for Me?"

It is clear that incoming generations of colleagues in medicine work differently, and make different choices than their senior colleagues on how they spend their time and energy. It is wonderful that new generations are more aware than ever of the need and importance of balancing their work and home lives, and of making time for their family and themselves. They do not seem satisfied with the services provided by workplace organizations, and see little value for their fees or time committed. However, the issues of the workplace will continue, and will require a continued forum to address and manage them.

For years now, the traditional organizations have struggled with declining membership, waning influence, and the need for new relevance for continued solvency. Medical organizations will need new innovative ways to attract memberships, and reverse this trend.

PERFORMANCE ENHANCEMENT

I have suggested to colleagues at the OPA that we take a page from the City of Ottawa, and try its methods that worked to recruit my twin sons recently. They were too old to go to the usual summer camps or have a sitter; but too young to get a job. My suggestion that they attend a City of Ottawa summer Leadership Camp was met by rolling eyes and shoulder shrugs. Since they had not actually said "No," I sent away for the brochure. I showed it to the boys when it arrived. On the cover was a picture of a boy about their age, with a bubble over his head, in which were written the words "I thought it would suck, but it didn't." It caught their attention—their sentiments exactly! They eventually called some of their friends, and as a group of six, they decided to try it out, with great success. To date, a picture of me talking about the OPA with a similar word bubble has not been approved by Council!

Seriously—we will need to work on identifying the issues that will motivate people to come out and work together. There is no need to create a crisis; there are plenty of them within medicine to identify and work together to resolve. As well, testimonials from colleagues already involved help make others consider doing the same. We will need to gather this information, and then make it known to our junior colleagues. The added value of working with colleagues from other parts of the city, province, or country is wonderful. The sense of collegiality and the opportunity to network is a draw. Such involvement offers a chance to gain and strengthen administrative skills. Many colleagues appreciate the opportunity to advocate for patients as a group, and make things happen that are not possible to do on one's own.

I know that the main reason that I have become involved with medical organizations is because of a personal touch. Someone I know, like, and admire is always the instigator—they ask me to get involved, and I appreciate and accept the opportunity to work with them. Then, I am consistently impressed by how much fun and productive it actually turns out to be. It worked for me, and is the reason I make the time to phone or email others personally.

SECTION SIX

As I make this call, I know that even if I can't think of any thing else to say, I can always tell them "I thought it would suck, but it didn't!"

Successfully Managing Your Career in Medicine

We have all taken a distinct path to becoming a physician. Some of us knew from the very start that this is what we wanted to be when we grew up. Others knew once we started high school. Still others among us had no idea what we wanted to do even when we were at university. Regardless of when we decided, we were all mostly so excited to be in medical school, and even more excited to graduate, that we gave little thought to what it was going to be like to practice medicine every day. In fact, the average physician finishes medical school in their mid-to-late-20's, and retires in their mid-to-late-60's. That gives us about 40 working years to fill...and hopefully, enjoy. It used to be that doctors finished their training, and expected to practice medicine for the rest of their lives, and then retire. Such a career trajectory is uncommon these days. Luckily, there is a lot of choice to allow us to successfully manage our career in medicine.

One of my mentors in medical school shared with me his Seven-Year Rule, his belief that we can only do, and enjoy what we are doing, for about seven years at a time. He encouraged me to regularly reassess what I was doing every seven years or so, and modify it so I could continue to appreciate and feel a sense of reward through my work. Inherent in this was a huge lesson— that a career is not something that just happens to me, that the key to career satisfaction is to proactively shape my own career path.

There are three well-described stages of any career. The first stage is when we have the most energy and drive, feel full of excitement and enthusiasm, and feel ready to set bold goals and work to achieve them. Possibilities seem endless during this time. When we hit the second stage, reality sets in. We start to realize that we may not be able to do it all. It becomes harder to remain focused on the original goals and we may start to feel tired or discouraged. In the third stage of our career, we redefine our goals and priorities and reconcile our decisions. We set new accessible goals, see challenges ahead that we can meet, and work towards that, with success. These stages occur within a medical career, too. Being aware of this allows us to monitor and react effectively when we reach a new stage.

I just attended my 25th medical school reunion last fall. It was great to reflect over the years, and see the range of what we were all doing. Some of my classmates continued to practice clinical medicine primarily, but others had added educational, administrative, or research duties. We were all abuzz about a colleague who left medicine after 15 years of practice to become a makeup artist on Broadway. We spoke of loving our work, of finding it meaningful, of feeling overwhelmed and burnt out, of being too busy and out of balance, of realizing that medicine was not the right fit for us, of having the opportunity of doing something else now that the kids were grown up, or of just wanting to do something else now. Despite a variety of reasons, all of us were ready for some change. Fortunately, such change can easily occur within medicine, allowing us to make the required adjustments so we can feel more fulfilled.

It is crucial to realize that stages of career development are normal, natural, necessary, and will occur. Over the next few chapters, I will take a closer look at this process. We will explore it from a temporal point of view—before, during, and after the change. In the next chapter, we will look at the process before we even take any steps, understanding the reasons to make a change, and anticipating potential barriers to this. Next, we will discuss how to consider and choose options that may work for us. In the final instalment, we will identify practical steps towards our new direction, and address how we can best deal with the change.

Being a physician is both a calling and a career. Career development is lifelong and occurs throughout the major stages of our life. Managing our career in medicine is an important skill to develop and cultivate, and is a process that we each must actively lead for ongoing career satisfaction.

PERFORMANCE ENHANCEMENT

Career Development: Assessment & Exploration

Medicine has been a rich and rewarding career. Yet, lately, you have started to feel restless, recognizing that work seems to be less stimulating and challenging than it used to be. This is not uncommon; the majority of us will experience this at some point in our career. To recapture the initial sense of excitement about coming to work each morning, there will be some important decisions to make ahead. We are well trained to make decisions for our patients when they present with a medical problem; the same process of analysis applies here. We need to analyze the situation so we can understand it; identify and explore options; choose an option and create a plan of action; and then implement it and evaluate the outcome.

First, let's understand why we want a change. There are many reasons why we desire a change in our current work situation. These include:

Burnout; We may be feeling overloaded and realizing that our workload and responsibilities are not sustainable.

Work place issues; We are not happy in the work environment, or with the people we work.

Frustration with health care system; It is increasingly more difficult to practice medicine with decreased resources, increased workloads, more regulations and limitations, and rising malpractice rates.

Wrong original choice; Some of us chose medicine because it was the right thing to do, what our parents hoped we would do, or what our school guidance teachers recommended for us. We may have selected a specialty that does not suit us well. It may not be the best fit for us.

Seven-year itch; Many of us start to feel bored with what we are doing after several years and need a change.

New interests; Our interests have expanded and changed, and we would like our work to reflect this.

Need for more stimulation; The job is good enough, but is not exciting or challenging any more. It feels like the same old thing each day.

Financial freedom; We have paid our debts, the kids are through university, and we now have gained financial freedom to not work the way we used to do. Alternatively, we want a different job that may offer us greater financial freedom that our current practice.

Life changes; Marriage, marital separation, having children, empty nest syndrome, dealing with aging parents—all may cause us to reassess our work.

Health problems; We may have a health problem that limits our energy and our capacity to work in the way we did previously.

Once we identify some of the reasons to consider a change, we start to see why the change seems impossible. There are many barriers to such a change for many of us:

Guilt; We have a huge sense of responsibility to our patients, staff, and family. How can we do this to them?

Shame; There is a sense of shame, that we will be perceived as being unable to cope, that we "couldn't cut it" in medicine.

Fear of failure; What if we don't succeed after the change? Too many people seem to be depending on us, and we can't let them down.

Finances; We can't afford to stop practicing medicine. There are few other things we can do that offer the same pay per hour so consistently, and so we often stay because the money is good.

Uncertainty; We may not know what the options are, or where to go for advice.

PERFORMANCE ENHANCEMENT

Over the years, I have come up with the Three-Step Rule for career change:

1. Modify.

2. Change within medicine.

3. Change outside of medicine.

There are times when we know what exactly we want to do and go for it. However, more often, there is no perfect or quick solution, and it helps to take it one step at a time. In many situations, things improve with modifying the current practice—reassessing the work hours, changing the location of the practice or joining a new group, changing the scope of practice, or balancing work with a non-medical activity. If this is insufficient, then you can consider defining a new focus within medicine. Such career diversification can include medical education, leadership, administration, or research roles. Finally, we could explore roles outside medicine where our medical skills and knowledge would be welcomed, such as with the government, a medical organization, an insurance company, a pharmaceutical company, computers and technology, consulting, writing, and speaking; or even new roles not connected to medicine at all.

The process starts with a review and reflection of your current situation. Identify what you now like and dislike about work, your values, your future goals, elements that you would like to have at work, your skills and strengths and weaknesses, your interests and fears, what you are deeply passionate about, and at what you can be the best. You can start this on your own. There are some career counselling books that can guide this process. Some colleagues find it helpful to work with a career counsellor, advisor, or coach.

We can now start to develop a career focus and explore career options. We look around and see what our colleagues may be doing, and find out what potential positions exist. We can turn to resources such as books, websites, and job search groups. Like building a custom home, we look at what possibilities have all of what we need, most of what we want, and some of the fun parts, too. It helps to be specific, take your time, and give it a lot of thought. As we picture the ideal first month on the job, we have a good idea of where we may want to go. In the next chapter, we will look at how to get there.

Career Development: Deciding & Moving Forward

Many of us reach that point when we know that a change in the course of our medical career is inevitable.

We may have decided to modify our current medical practice. We can reassess the number or range of hours we work, move to a different practice location, or move to work with new colleagues. We can look at our scope of practice, and identify and eliminate what we no longer enjoy about our practice (e.g., choose to stop doing obstetrics in our family practice) or balance it with some positive medical or non-medical activity (e.g., free up a half day to take art classes). This may just bring us the positive change we seek.

Sometimes, we choose to define a new focus in medicine. This may mean pursuing further training to change the clinical focus of our work, such as completing a one-year fellowship to do GP Anesthesia, or learning to use lasers in our practice. In fact, doctors in clinical medicine occupy only about one percent of the workforce; there are so many other things we can do. Further career diversification can include options such as adding on roles in medical education, leadership, administration, and research. As well, remember that there are also many roles possible outside medicine.

Making a change in our careers in mid-life is not easy. Generally, the higher up the ladder one is, the harder it is to choose something different as there is more one has to lose. However, if you are truly not happy, every day that you stay is another day that you fall behind. It is important to do what you love, but one does need to have proper financial and business plans. It helps to have a financial cushion before you leap. A mentor of mine often suggests that colleagues put away money from the start of their career, so as to support a possible year "off" fifteen years later.

There are several factors to consider in the timing of a career change. Clear earning expectations should be defined; there is often a decrease in income since there are relatively few other positions that offer the consistently high earnings we enjoy in medicine. We need to have a sense of clarity and focus. The size of our network may be a factor, as is the time and the money we have to invest in this change. We need to consider our own willingness to relocate, as well as the support we would have from our partner and family. It helps to know and understand our past history and experiences with change, as this will enter into this current experience, too.

There is great discussion about whether one should go back to school. Education is crucial, and qualifications are necessary. Yet, more is not better. You can highlight the formal education you already have, and transferable skills you have gained; and future employers already know that you can learn. If you do decide to get further education, do so with a sense of clear purpose, and begin with the end in mind.

Once we have taken a full assessment of our interests, skills, values, and goals, we can create a vision of our future. We enter a phase of career exploration, in which we need to explore what is available in this area, update our CV, research potential employers, prepare for interviews, and explore work environments and colleagues. Next is the decision making stage, where we can narrow down choices, make a decision and develop a game plan. At this point, we can let others know if our plans through networking, letters, and personal meetings, so they can support us. We are off to a new beginning.

PERFORMANCE ENHANCEMENT

Career Development: Logical Next Steps & Dealing with Change

So, we have now decided that we want to change some aspect of our career in medicine. We must have a clear understanding about our selves, and why we want this change.

What is the logical next step? Whatever we do, it must make sense, and be understandable in light of where we are and where we want to go. There are some practical strategies we can use as we move forward. If we have decided to focus on a new aspect of medicine, we can start to go to conferences in that area of interest. There are specialized journals, publications, and books we can read. We can take a course on this topic. There is plenty to browse through on the internet, and you can even create your own related website. We can join an association, start networking, get a mentor. A great way to show others that you are interested and capable is to volunteer in a related capacity; by taking on extra responsibility, you can demonstrate your dedication and willingness and help them to see you as a potential resource.

For big changes, a good rule is the "80% to 20% overlap," in which you initiate a change by maintaining 80% of your current activities, while 20% of what you do should be new, different, exciting, and fun. Whenever possible, try not to make a complete change all at once. This gives you time to adjust and confirm that the change is what you want. Set a realistic timeline; it usually takes two to three years for a major transition.

Dealing with change, even if it is a change that we chose and want, is not easy. Changing or closing a clinical practice is truly difficult and draining, and we always underestimate the associated emotional and physical toll. There is a lot of work to do, charts to complete, summaries to write, transfers to facilitate. There is a sense of loss, by our patients, our colleagues, and our self. Part of dealing with a loss is allowing for the stages of grieving—denial, anger and protest, bargaining, sadness, acceptance, and integration. This is physically and emotionally exhausting, even when we expect it. While dealing with the denial, anger, and protest is not easy, many of us are surprised to realize it is also not easy to receive the kindness and gratitude that is expressed at this time by patients, their families, colleagues, and friends. I recall receiving compliments, praise, and even small tokens of appreciation as I reduced my clinical work. It was a very touching and emotional process. It can be overwhelming, making us feel guilty, and even making us question if we are making the right decision. Ultimately, it is helpful to remind yourself regularly why you chose this transition and what good lies ahead

"I am not a doctor anymore." If the decision we make involves giving up clinical medical practice entirely, many of us initially find it tough to consider no longer being a doctor. This has been a huge part of our identity. There is an associated status, prestige, and sense of recognition with this occupation, which we now feel at risk of losing. There can be an awareness of ageing, of having to face our mortality. This can seem challenging and even scary. However, the reality is that we will always be a doctor. We will always have the training and education, and will be utilizing them in a new manner to maintain our skills, expertise, knowledge, and attitude.

It is up to us to actively shape our career paths. In doing so in a positive, proactive manner, we can continue to set future goals and continue to mature personally and professionally, and enjoy satisfying careers.

SECTION SEVEN

MAINTAINING YOUR PEAK PERFORMANCE: RESILIENCY IN MEDICINE

·

How Resilient Are You?

I have worked with physicians in distress for years. Interventions with physicians have been based primarily on pathology: identifying, responding to, and solving problems. More recently, I started to look at physician health from a different perspective, and ask "Why do some physicians cope better than others in the same situation?" Some of them seemed to have more resilience. Yet that led to more questions. What is resilience? What are the qualities of a resilient physician? What was it about them—is it a way of thinking? A way of doing? Was it something they just had in them? Could it be taught? This new focus on resilience is proactive, positive, and offers primary prevention. It helps to recognize strengths and skills, and offers an opportunity to develop strategies for success that build on existing capabilities.

Resilience is a word often used, yet it can mean different things to different people. The more I researched this, the more I recognized that we do not really have a full definition of this concept. There is not much written on this topic, and each author has a distinct view. Perhaps all the various definitions are part of the complete picture, and resilience has many dimensions. My goal is to clarify and define this further.

The American Psychological Association, post-9/11, defined resilience as "the ability to adapt well in the face of adversity, trauma, tragedy, threats, and from sources of stress such as work pressures, health, family, or relationship problems."

In my practice, I have seen how possessing resilience allows people to bounce back, and rebound from major life setbacks even stronger than before. Healthy people with a lot of resilience have personalities that seem resistant to stress, and can learn valuable lessons from difficult experiences. They are confident and optimistic. In tough situations, while they may feel under-standably distressed, they assume that things will work out well in some way. They have a reaction that is focused on coping and learning, rather than being a victim and blaming.

MAINTAINING YOUR PEAK PERFORMANCE

As physicians, there are so many stressors we deal with on a daily basis in all parts of our lives. Some of them are inherent to our work, as we take care of others and intimately witness fellow humans suffer and meet life's challenges.

We also have to deal with changes and transitions in our own life. Medical training brings with it the stressors at each phase— medical school, starting clinical work, graduation, residency training, and early career issues as we set up practice, consider later career adjustments and changes, and then plan for retirement. There are associated financial stressors. There are physical moves, to new hospitals, neighborhoods, cities, and even countries. We all experience ongoing changes with our personal physical and mental health, and may have to learn to live with serious and chronic illnesses. There can be personal transitions, including dating, marriage, separation, and divorce. We may have children, and deal with the various challenges at each phase of their lives, and then deal with the empty nest as they grow up and move away. Some of us deal with issues of infertility, and consider options of treatment and adoption, or adjusting to a life without children. Life brings loss, and we deal with the serious illness and death of loved ones—parents, partners, friends, colleagues, and children. In other countries of the world, physicians deal with all of this, as well as managing the devastating results of hunger, poverty, or war.

Resilience is the ultimate life skill.

According to the Harvard Business Review, 2002, "...more than education, more than experience, more than training, an individual's level of resilience will determine who succeeds and who fails."

I believe that resilience can be taught so we can better succeed. There are some non-modifiable factors, such as our genetics, parents, upbringing, and childhood experiences that play a role in our current abilities to cope through difficult situations. Yet, there are many modifiable factors, too. We can learn to modify our perceptions of our self and the situation, recognize learned behaviours and assumptions that do not help us, attain a positive attitude, become more self assertive and set limits and boundaries, and be more confident in reaching out and connecting with others.

Resilient Doctors Are Confident Doctors

Resilience is the ability to deal with difficult events, be flexible and bounce back, and grow as a result. It is a dynamic concept, an ongoing process which can vary over time. It has many dimensions, including a sense of confidence and control which will be the focus of this chapter.

Confident people are those who have a positive view of themselves, their strengths and their abilities, and are known to cope better during stressful situations. Developing such confidence and nurturing a positive view of one self is possible, and helps build resilience.

Where does this self image come from? Our sense of self is the product of learning, built though our life experiences since early childhood. The greatest contribution comes during our formative years, from parents and caregivers who serve as mirrors and reflect back to us an image of ourselves. Experiences with other family members, teachers, and friends add to the information we use to create our self image. It is reinforced by messages from the media, as well as ongoing relationships and experiences. These are integrated to create an inner sense of our strengths, weaknesses, physical appearance, values, and adequacy. This is what I call the Historian, a teller of our personal history. If it is positive, we can appreciate our assets and potential, and be realistic about our limitations. It can help us see accept change, focus on what we can control, and conceptualize challenges as opportunities to learn and grow. Yet, if negative, we focus on our faults and distort imperfections, and minimize or even dismiss abilities and achievements. This influences how we think about ourselves, which in turn, influences our behaviour and how we react to stressful events.

Many doctors have had childhood experiences they have perceived as providing negative feedback, which has led to a sense of personal inadequacy, of not measuring up. This is an unconscious conclusion, and while we are not aware of it, it impacts our behaviour. It is part of the reason for our success to date—it leads us to try harder, do better, and achieve more. Yet, the Historian often continues to perpetuate the feelings of inadequacy. We are not always able to feel confident in our abilities and achievements, and may have a persistent sense of self-doubt. We feel like an impostor, even though there is no basis to this. While we can appreciate this when our friends and colleagues do it, and tell them it is not true, we cannot see how we do it ourselves. Try the "Best Friend" technique—when feeling negative about yourself, think of your best friends feeling down on themselves for no reason, and what you may say to them. Then, say the same to yourself.

I believe that we are all born with a positive sense of self, and imagine it to be like a shiny bright jewel. Just look at children in healthy environments, innocently taking pride in what they do and celebrating simple accomplishments. I recall one of my sons at age two, climbing up onto the piano bench, randomly striking piano keys, then clapping his hands and taking a bow. His positive sense of self was apparent, glowing like a gem. If I were to reply "Good job," the jewel would continue to glow. Yet, had I told him to "quit making that noise," or to "climb down from that bench before he fell off," I would have put a layer over that gem and it would shine a little less brightly. Repeated negative incidents put more layers on the jewel, so that it becomes less visible and then forgotten. Over time, we may become self-critical, adding layers ourselves when no one else is doing so.

Luckily, we can learn to rewrite our history so it is more accurate and less distorted. Cognitive therapy can assist with this. We learn to recognize how we distort our thinking, challenge our negative self-attitudes and self-perceptions, and balance them with positive self affirmation. Effectively, we catch ourselves as we start to add a layer of covering and stop. We can even learn to unwrap previous layers, and slowly, start to see the jewel shining through again.

While self confidence is an attitude that we can develop, this takes time; there is no quick fix. There are two aspects of this—

self esteem, and self efficacy—both of which must be reinforced. Self esteem is the sense that we have strengths and can cope with what is going on in our life. Self efficacy is our competence, our ability to learn knowledge and master skills, so that we can accept challenges, persist, and succeed. With the right combination of attitude and knowledge, in a time of stress or crisis, the confident person is optimistic and has the sense and belief that they can do it. As a colleague recently told me during an exceptionally stressful time, "While I don't want to be going through this, I don't question that I can."

A positive self worth fosters personal growth through adversity. There is freedom from doubt, leaving no question that, in any situation, we will handle what is presented, and succeed.

SECTION SEVEN

Resilient Doctors Are Connected Doctors

In my training as a child psychiatrist, I recall reading with great interest about Donald Winnicott's conceptualization of the psychic space between the mother and child, which he termed the Holding Environment. If this were properly created and provided by the mother, it allowed for the child to feel "held"—taken care of, safe, protected, understood, loved. This formed the basis for the child to learn to trust and grow, and transition to becoming more autonomous. In fact, I realize that we need nourishing "holding environments" throughout our life, so we can continue to feel safe and grow. As we get older, these holding environments build resiliency, and can be found within the context of our school, sports teams, friendships, relationships, and in our workplace. The key aspect of the holding environment is the presence of people who make us feel held.

The single most powerful predictor of resilience is the presence of caring connections with others. We need to create these relationships, and then reach out to them regularly for help, support, guidance, and encouragement.

The culture of medicine makes this crucial aspect of connecting difficult to attain. In our training, we are taught to be tough and strong, and to manage on our own. If our past experiences in life have taught us that there is little help available and we can only count on ourselves, we survive well in medicine where this is the norm. We have full practices and busy days, focus on providing our best care, and often do not have time to stop and socialize with colleagues. Even if we did have time, many hospitals have now done away with the traditional doctors' lounge, a place where much of the conversations and connections were created and maintained. Ironically, many prestigious research universities are now busy creating "convergence" areas, bringing together experts and students from multiple disciplines to work on a single research topic—and they deliberately mix the cafeteria, lounge, and library area in order to foster those conversations that lead to "Aha" moments.

MAINTAINING YOUR PEAK PERFORMANCE

A study of life satisfaction and resilience in Norwegian medical schools (Kjeldstadli, Tyssen, et al, published in BMC Medical education, 2006) concluded that medical schools should encourage students to maintain their outside interests, friends, and personal lives. Jensen, Trollope-Kumar, and associates in Hamilton, Canada, explored dimensions of family physician resilience (Canadian Family Physician, 2008 May), and highlighted the value of supportive relations, which include positive personal relationships, professional relationships, and good communication. Yet another study by Lemaire and Wallace (*On Physician Wellbeing: You'll get by with a little help from your friends*, 2005) showed that support from spouses and coworkers, as well as positive patient interactions is a key factor to reduce stress and increase wellbeing.

In our professional life, we must look for opportunities to build positive relationships—with our colleagues, medical team, staff, and patients. Doctors tell me that one of the biggest stresses at work is working with other doctors who are stressed. Take time to get to know your colleagues, find out a bit about them as people, ask about people, things and events that are important to them. Attend and join in social activities in the workplace. Be positive and appreciative to others; look for good things daily and comment on them. Enjoy the opportunities and privilege our patients offer by allowing us into their lives at pivotal times. Look for and be a mentor. Create a culture of collaboration and collegiality, learn to communicate effectively, and resolve conflict in a healthy manner. Make time to sit down with peers, talk about difficult cases, and offer support. Many doctors speak of the value of their journal club, small learning groups, or Balint groups. I can personally attest to how my journal club has bolstered my ability to be resilient. Our group (we call ourselves the PALS—Psychiatrists At Large!) has been meeting monthly for about 20 years. They are the perfect holding environment— they are reliably present, make me feel liked and respected, and so allow me to ask questions and advice without fear of being seen as weak/stupid/failing. While we have greatly contributed to ensuring we are all medically up to date, we have also seen, supported, and celebrated each other as we go through life and all that it has to offer.

In our personal life, all of us require a personal support system of partner, family, friends, and social and spiritual community. A supportive home environment allows us to recharge at the end of a busy day, and creates energy so we can go back and do it again the next day. Such an environment must be constantly nurtured. We need to allocate meaningful time for this, to make and keep regular dates with our significant others, family, and friends. We have to be available and present when we are not at work, to participate actively in life at home. Regular communication is essential with the people we care about. Some people find that being active in community, civic, or faith-based organizations provide social support.

The primary factor in resilience is having caring and supportive relationships in all parts of our life. Relationships that create love and trust, provide positive role models, and offer encouragement and reassurance provide a buffer against adversity and help us to build resilience. There is strength in numbers; the people around us make us strong. Make sure you create such relationships and reach out and use them!

A Resilient Doctor Is a Committed Doctor

As doctors, we choose to enter the medical profession because we want to make a difference. We can easily recall that dream we had as a medical student—of wanting to cure illness, stamp out disease, and make our patients better. Many of us affirmed this as we took the Hippocratic Oath, promising to uphold professional ethical standards as we treat patients with spirit, diligence, and dedication.

Having a continued sense of commitment to this cause allows us to face each day and persevere, especially at times when it is not always easy to do so. This commitment to what we value and respect is key to our ability to be resilient. As long as we can feel that we are living fully and working towards meaningful goals, we are able to manage with whatever is thrown our way.

In medicine, we must ask ourselves and constantly remember "What drew us to this?" As we start working, it is easy to become too busy and lose sight of what was initially meaningful to us. Medicine is both a calling and a career. Over the 40 years that the average physician works, we can go through many normal and natural phases of our career. In the early phase, we are still full of energy and excitement and anticipation, and have a lot of drive. This gives way to the middle phase, when the reality sets in, and we are not able to do all that we want to, and have to reframe our goals to fit our current reality. It is here that we may question our commitment to medicine, and so need to remain focused. The later phase follows, in which we define and reconcile our priorities, restate our commitments and forge ahead. One of my psychiatry professors wisely told me that we can only do what we are doing well for about seven years at a time; then we should reassess and modify it to continue to enjoy it. We must actively shape our career paths in medicine so we can continue to feel committed to work that we enjoy. While this is not easy, bringing up initial fears, guilt and uncertainties, it almost always results positively in a renewed sense of commitment.

SECTION SEVEN

Journaling is a way of telling and recalling our story. In her book, *Kitchen Table Wisdom: Stories that Heal*, Rachel Naomi Remen invites us to "listen from the soul." Her concept of Kitchen Table Wisdom is that of the human tradition of shared experiences and stories told around the kitchen table, which demonstrate life with all its power and mystery, and reminds us that the things we may not be able to measure may just be what ultimately enrich and sustain our lives. Try it yourself! Sit with a blank piece of paper, and reflect. Ask yourself what made you decide to become a doctor, what now gives you meaning as a doctor, what story stands out in your memory as the best thing you have ever done as a doctor. These stories will serve to accomplish what Dr. Remen encourages us to do—to "recapture the soul in medicine."

While a vital commitment to our work is essential, this is even better extended to all aspects of our life. Ideally, we commit to life, to living fully and aiming for meaningful personal and professional goals.

Viktor Frankl describes his experiences in the concentration camps in his book, *Man's Search For Meaning*, and explains how his sense of commitment to values and goals enabled him to survive such an experience. He created logotherapy, a form of psychotherapy which considers man as a "being whose main concern consists in fulfilling a meaning and in actualizing values, rather than in the mere gratification and satisfaction of drives and instincts…What man actually needs is not a tensionless state but rather the striving and struggling for some goal worthy of him. What he needs is not the discharge of tension at any cost, but the call of a potential meaning waiting to be fulfilled by him."

To be at our most resilient, we can identify the aspects that we value in all parts of our life—at work, relationships, family, home, friends, and for our self—and decide what we are going to do to maintain these priorities. Think of the story of the Big Rocks and the Little Rocks. A professor shows the class a pile of big rocks, small rocks, sand, and some water, and asks them how to put them all into a big bowl. If the water or sand go in first, there is not enough room for the rocks. Yet, if the big rocks go in first, the small rocks will all fit in around the bigger ones, and the sand will fill in among the rocks, and there is even room for the water in the bowl. The message is that the order of which we do things is crucial—that we place the big rocks in first. Identify what your Big Rocks (priorities) are, and place them in your day (bowl) first.

As we set, reassess, and reset personal and professional plans and goals, we can ensure they are realistic and meaningful, and will continue to provide us a sense of fulfillment and purpose. Once the things we do in our life make sense, we can more easily cope with the challenges along the way, and sustain the sense of wisdom, wonder, and richness of life.

SECTION SEVEN

A Resilient Doctor Is a Calm Doctor

We all know them—the doctors who can be in the midst of turbulence and chaos, and manage to stay calm. These are the colleagues at work whom we admire, since their day seems to take less out of them. We wonder how they do it, as we become increasingly frustrated and reactive. As physicians working in highly complex situations, challenges seem to occur daily; and it is normal to have resultant thoughts, feelings, and emotions. Yet, the behaviour that can result form such negative emotions is unhealthy for us, and often unacceptable for others.

There are basically two factors in being calm:

- Learning how to recognize triggers and when things are starting to build up.
- Developing successful strategies for managing the associated emotions.

During a quiet moment, take time to reflect what the triggers are, both at home and at work. There is usually something or someone that pushes our buttons. Think about this, and try to understand the inherent patterns. In a previous chapter on resilience, we spoke about my 90:10 Rule, that only 10% of our reaction in any situation comes from that specific situation, 90% is from past experiences. Try to acknowledge this, and dial down the intensity of reaction to a tenth of what you feel at that moment. This allows you to stay calmer, and use one or more of the techniques below to maintain your sense of calm and control, and cope more easily.

None of us does it perfectly. It helps to have a range of tools to rely on as needed. Just as we want to have a spectrum of antibiotics to use, choosing depending on factors such as the site and organism causing the infection; when we know of a range of techniques to calm ourselves, we can more easily choose and access the best one for that situation.

Take a deep breath. This is a good first choice, as it is easy to remember, takes little time, gives you a chance to stop and not just react, allows you to focus on something else for a moment, and provides extra oxygen to your brain while you are thinking of how to respond.

Count to ten. This is easy, distracting, and again, it buys you a bit of time before you start to react to the situation.

Reframing. How we think impacts how we feel; this is the basic underlying premise of cognitive therapy. A good example is the concept of Recalculating. As our car's GPS tell us when we take a wrong turn or go off course unexpectedly, it is "recalculating" and comes up with a new plan of action. Yet, it does so in a calm, unemotional, non-judgmental manner. In my home, we have taken on this phrase to remind and encourage each other to "recalculate" similarly when things go off course unexpectedly.

Positivity. Research shows a clear link between positive emotions and a happy, healthy, and productive life. Consciously look for the good in the world around you, make a positive contribution yourself, express appreciation, and be optimistic.

Relaxation Exercises. There are so many different exercises to help us relax after our bodies deal with tension. These work to break down the tension, relax the muscles, and promote an over-all relaxed physical and emotional state. They create a relaxation response, a state of deep rest. Relaxation techniques can include active or passive progressive muscular relaxation, visualization, and yoga. Find music or a CD/DVD that can guide you properly through such an exercise.

Mindfulness Meditation. Meditation helps to increase our awareness of our reactions and to develop healthier ways to cope. By staying in the present moment, and facing problems, we can reflect, gain a new perspective, and manage and act differently. We focus on observing our breath, thoughts, feelings, and sensation; experience what is actually happening instead of ruminating or trying to change things. We often see more possibilities, instead of reacting in our usual patterns of behaviour.

SECTION SEVEN

Nurture Spirituality. Spirituality is defined as the deepest values and meanings by which one lives. Spiritual practices focus on developing our inner life, thereby allowing us to feel more connected with, and have faith in, the world around us. Having faith has been shown to give one strength and comfort. Spirituality is not the same as religion, but religion can be one form of spirituality.

Journaling. Taking time to put feeling into words helps clarify things and highlight options not previously seen. When writing, we can have an outlet and let go of feelings that we cannot or should not share with others. Writing about a difficult day at work, or a tragic patient outcome, allows us to validate and manage our feelings in a safe, private, and effective manner.

Any of the previous techniques can be effective in assisting us to feel a sense of calm at home and at work, but we have to practice. It is a process of learning and teaching our body what a calm state feels like and how to attain it. The more we do it, the easier it becomes. When practiced regularly, these activities will lead to a reduction in daily stress levels and an increase in sense of joy and calmness. They serve as protective armour in the face of life's challenges, and give us the strength and energy to remain resilient.

MAINTAINING YOUR PEAK PERFORMANCE

A Resilient Physician Cares for Self

Caring for others is inherent in being a physician. This is what we do best—it is intuitive for us, we are trained to do this, and it is our role and goal. Having empathy for others, a desire to care for others and make a difference in their lives, and the ability and capability to do so enable us to be resilient. It provides a sense of meaning to our work, which helps to ground us during times of stress and crisis. Yet, caring for others is not enough; to be sustainable, it must be balanced with caring for our self.

Caring for our self is often less intuitive and definitely not part of our training. It is not our role—we are care givers, not care receivers. Thus, it is no surprise that this is not easy for us to do consistently. We put our own needs last, and often, they are lost.

A large aspect of self care is taking care of our physical health. We are the only ones who can ensure that we eat properly, sleep long enough and restoratively, exercise regularly, keep our brains active, and have a family doctor and see him/her regularly. We can also monitor our emotional health, knowing and watching out for the signs of burnout. It is crucial to identify our priorities, both at work and at home, and to regularly reflect on how well we are doing at making time for all of them. Taking care of ourselves also includes things like taking time to relax, indulging our self, making time for personal hobbies, spending time with people that we enjoy, laughing, taking regular holidays and time off work. Once you find activities that you enjoy which make you feel relaxed and replenished, use the Tarzan Rule to keep them going; do not stop and let go of a positive activity until you have one more booked! That way, you know it is going to happen again.

Interestingly, I find that when colleagues do have or make some time for themselves, it's been so long since the last time… they often do not know what to do with it! The first time you have a bit of free time, you may need to stop and think about what you would do the next time that happens. Take time for yourself proactively. Ask yourself:

- If I had the afternoon off to do whatever I wanted, I would…
- I remember years ago when I would love to…
- I would be really disappointed if I never get to…
- Something I have always wanted to try is…
- I would love to spend more time with…

Reflect on these answers, and look for a way to make this happen now.

All of this requires that we give our self permission to care for our self. As a group of professionals, we are very conscientious and responsible, and often feel guilty when we are not working. We see time for ourselves as a luxury, as being selfish and focusing on ourselves when there is so much else to do. In fact, this is an investment—if you take a small amount of time and energy for yourself, you are much more likely to be available to those who count on you. Remember the airline safety demonstration—in the case of an emergency, you are advised to put on your own oxygen mask first before you assist someone else. You are no good to anyone else if you pass out! This is an excellent reminder for our work in medicine; we have to stop and do the metaphorical equivalent of putting our own masks on first, especially in times of stress or crisis.

While it is understandable to feel guilty, this is not necessary. Self care is not an either/or proposition. Imagine a bubble full of the names of all the people (family, friends, patients, colleagues, community) that we care for and about. Just "open this bubble" and put your own name in there, too. No one will miss the small amount of time and energy they do not get as a result, but taking a tiny sliver from everyone will create a nice portion for your self.

Think of your dream car—bold, beautiful, powerful, a pleasure to drive. Imagine that you have bought it, and driven it every chance you had for a couple of weeks…then it runs out of gas and comes to a halt. It does not matter how much potential it has; unless it has fuel, it is going nowhere! We are exactly the same. Despite our potential, we also need fuel to keep going. Unfortunately, unlike cars, we do not come with a gas gauge. We need to monitor this ourselves on an ongoing basis, and making a conscious effort to "Top Up Our Tank™" in a proactive manner. This will ensure that we have the energy needed to go the distance, manage during the stress, remain resilient, and bounce back stronger and wiser.

SECTION SEVEN

Resilient Physicians Deserve Resilient Medical Systems

Attempting to define the dimensions of resilience in physicians in past chapters has been an enriching experience. Instead of answers, my questions often led to more questions. The five components that I have defined are a good start, informed by years of clinical experience. Yet, it is clear that this area is one that requires much more thought and research in the future.

There will always be stress in the practice of medicine. Much of this is positive, healthy, and motivating. The desirable goal in assisting physicians to become more resilient is to have them build skills and energy reserves so they can continue to cope well in times of stress. Young's modulus, from engineering's solid mechanics, refers to the measure of the stiffness of an isotropic elastic material. It refers to the ratio of stress, with units of pressure, to strain. In medicine, while we are hoping to reduce the strain, we have no real units of pressure to measure the stress. As well, the stress comes from multiple sources, and varies depending on the physician, their specialty, and demographics; thus it requires multiple resources to manage.

Addressing the five components of resilience in an individual physician is like laminating a piece of paper. It gives it an extra coat, makes it hardier, and more flexible. It will allow the physician to feel more empowered and confident to handle unforeseen and unpredictable events, and so can enhance the system. Yet, it is not enough.

I recently had a thought-provoking discussion with a colleague in the Department of Epidemiology on the value of improving resilience among colleagues. Is this a good thing? Or can this be exploitative? The concern, of course, is that as the situation in medicine continues to worsen with fewer resources and more stressors, we merely respond by helping doctors just cope better and do more with less. Doctors are known to be responsible, conscientious, and people-pleasing; and are not good at demonstrating "visible pain." When things are tough, and there is more to do, we just buckle down and do more. The end result is that we take on the pain, yet it is not visible to others who just assume that everything is fine. The irony is that unless others see the pain, there is nothing for them to respond to and improve to lessen the pain. Thus, the system does not improve. What we are striving for is a balance, one in which physicians feel more empowered to cope in difficult situations, and also have a voice and sense of control to make their pain visible, to constructively identify the problems that need to be addressed and resolved.

It is clear that making physicians more resilient cannot occur in isolation. The relationship between physician and systemic resilience is complex, and bi-directional. While we can assist the individual physician to proactively manage in a healthier manner, we need system level interventions too. The goal is not to train our physicians to merely become more plastic peons in the medical system. Resilient physicians require and deserve a more resilient medical system in which to work.

Bibliography

Books

Anderson, K., & MacSkimming, R. *On Your Own Again: The Down-to-Earth Guide to Getting Through a Divorce or Separation and Getting on with Your Life*. Toronto: McClelland & Stewart. 2007.

Boulis, Ann & Jacobs, Jerry. *The Changing Face of Medicine: Women Doctors and the Evolution of Health Care in America*. Ithatca and London: ILR Press, 2008.

Bridges, William. *Transitions: Making Sense of Life's Changes, 2nd Edition*. Cambridge: Da Capo Press, 1980.

Carnegie, Dale. *How to Win Friends and Influence People*. New York: Gallery Books, 1936.

Cohen, S., and Syme, S. *Social Support and Health*. New York: New York Academic Press, 1985.

Frankl, Viktor. *Man's Search for Meaning*. Boston: Beacon Press, 1959.

Fry, William. *Mirth and the Human Cardiovascular System: The Study of Humor*. Los Angeles: Antioch University Press, 1979.

Gautam, Mamta. *Irondoc*. Ottawa: Book Coach Press, 2005.

Holland, Barbara. *One's Company: Reflections on Living Alone*. Pleasantville: Arkadine Press, 1996.

Klaus, Peggy. *Brag! The Art of Tooting Your Own Horn without Blowing It*. New York: Warner Business Books, 2003.

Kriegel, R., & Brandt, D. *Sacred Cows Make the Best Burgers: Developing Change Ready People and Organizations*. New York: Warner Books, 1997.

Maslach, Christina. *The Maslach Burnout Inventory*. California: Mind Garden Inc, 1996.

Murdoch, Jeannie. *The Every Excuse in the Book Book: How to Benefit from Exercising by Overcoming Your Excuses*. BeanFit, 2005.

Parrott, Les and Leslie. *A Good Friend: 10 Traits of Enduring Ties*. Servant Publications, 1998.

Remen, Rachel Naomi. *Kitchen Table Wisdom: Stories that Heal*. New York: Riverhead Trade, 1997.

Journals & Publications

Annscheutz, B.L. "The high cost of caring...coping with workplace stress." *OACAS Journal* 43(3) (1999): 17-21.

Berk, Lee, et al. "Neuroendocrine and Stress Hormone Changes During Mirthful Laughter." *American Journal of the Medical Sciences* 298(6), (1989).

Bluestone, Naomi. "The Future Impact of Women on American Medicine." *American Journal of Public Health* 68, (1978): 760-763.

Cacioppo, John, & Hawkley, Louise. "Social Isolation and Health, with an Emphasis on Underlying Mechanisms." *Perspectives in Biology and Medicine*, vol. 46 (3), (2003): 39-52.

Frank, Erica et al. "Exercise Habits of Women Physicians." *JAMWA* 58, (2003): 178-184.

Klein, Laura et al. "Female Responses to Stress: Tend and Befriend, Not Fight or Flight." *Psychological Review*, 107 (3), (2000): 411-429.

Jensen, Trollope-Kumar et al. "Building Physician Resilience." *Canadian Family Physician* 54(5), (2008): 722-729.

Johnson, C.A. et al. "Perceived barriers to exercise and weight control practices in community women." *Women & Health* 16(3), (1990): 177-191.

Kjeldstadli, Tyssen, et al. "Life satisfaction and resilience in medical school." *BMC Medical Education* 6:48, (2006).

Putnam, Robert. "Bowling Alone: America's Declining Social Capital." *Journal of Democracy* 6(1), (1995): 65-78.

Seeman, Teresa et al. "Social Network Ties and Mortality Among Tile Elderly in the Alameda County Study." *American Journal of Epidemiology* 126, (1987):714-23.

Wallace, J., & Lemaire, J. "On Physician Wellbeing—You'll get by with a Little Help from your Friends." *Social Science & Medicine* 64, (2007): 2565-2577.

Williams et al. "Women in Medicine: practice patterns and attitudes." *Canadian Medical Association Journal* 143(3), (1990): 194-201.

Studies

Canadian Medical Association: *Physician Resource Questionnaire,* (2003).

Canadian Medical Protective Association: *Physician Survey,* (1996).

Harris County Medical Society Retired Physicians Organization: *Survey of Retired Physicians,* (1995).

Buckner, Dianne. *Seven Things that Women are not Told about Leadership*: CBC News World's Venture.

Elston, M.A. *Women and medicine: the future*: Royal College of Physicians, (2009).

Fooks, C., & Maxwell, J. *The Citizen's Dialogue: Future of Health Care in Canada*: Canadian Policy Research Networks, (2002).

Leeson et al. *The Future of Retirement in a World of Rising Life Expectancies*: HSBC, (2005).

Miller, Michael, *Laughter is Good for the Heart*: American Heart Association's 73rd Scientific Sessions, (2000).

ABOUT THE AUTHOR

Mamta Gautam, MD, FRCPC, CPDC is a psychiatrist in Ottawa, Canada, the author of *IronDoc,* and an Assistant Professor in the Department of Psychiatry at the University of Ottawa Faculty of Medicine. She is a visionary pioneer and specialist in Physician Health and Well-being. Hailed as "The Doctor's Doctor," physicians have made up her entire patient population for twenty years.

Dr. Gautam has an international reputation in the field of Physician Health, and all of her educational, administrative, and research activities have been focused in this area, leading its growth from a local to an international initiative. She is the founding Director of the University of Ottawa Faculty of Medicine Wellness Program, an innovative and comprehensive physician wellness program created in 2000, and which was the first of its kind at any academic setting in the world. This program served as the template for the national CMA Centre for Physician Health and Well-being, a concept she proposed in 2002, and where she has served as the Chair of the Expert Advisory Group, and as an expert Physician Advisor. She assisted in the creation of the Canadian Psychiatric Association Section on Physician Health, and served as the co-chair of this Section in its initial years. In 2008, she launched the International Alliance for Physician Health and was elected as the founding chair of this group.

Dr. Gautam is an internationally renowned expert and speaker. She has given over 1,000 keynote presentations and workshops in the area of physician stress and mental health, leadership in medicine, work-life balance in medicine, communication skills, and conflict resolution skills. She has authored numerous articles and book chapters on this topic, and created videos and pod-casts. She writes a regular column on

Physician Health, "Helping Hand," in the *Medical Post*; as well as a column, "Coach's Corner," in the *Newsletter of the Canadian Society of Physician Executives.*

In addition to her clinical work, Dr. Gautam founded PEAK MD in 2009, and serves as the President of this company which focuses on the expansion of her efforts in Physician Health to include primary prevention. This includes a greater focus on education and primary prevention workshops, as well as coaching physicians and physician leaders.

She is on the faculty of several medical leadership courses throughout Canada and the United States, including the Canadian Medical Association, Physician Manager Institute, Canadian Society of Physician Executives, and the Foundation for Medical Excellence. She also teaches professional resilience at the Telfer School of Management at the University of Ottawa, and the Schulich School of Business at York University.

Dr. Gautam has been awarded many honours for her work in Physician Health. Most recently, she was awarded the Canadian Medical Association's inaugural Physician Misericordia Award (2011), intended to recognize and celebrate physicians who have demonstrated outstanding leadership and support for their colleagues The College of Physicians and Surgeons of Ontario selected her as a 2004 Council Award recipient. This award "recognizes physicians who have demonstrated excellence, and come closest to meeting society's vision of an ideal physician." In both 2005 and 2006, she was nominated for a national award, the Canadian Workplace Wellness Pioneer Award, which recognizes an individual who has made a pioneering contribution to the field of organizational health. She was also a nominee for the 2005 YMCA-YWCA Women of Distinction Award for Healthy Living. This award recognizes women who have improved the well-being of their community and are outstanding leaders. The University of Ottawa awarded her the 2005 Alumni Award for Community Service to recognize her efforts on behalf of the medical community. She received an Honorary Fellowship in the

American Psychiatric Association in 2006, an honour awarded to a small select group of Canadian psychiatrists; and a Fellowship in the Canadian Psychiatric Association in 2007. She was nominated for the 2009 Indo-Canadian Ottawa Business Chamber Award, 2009 Women of Influence Award, and a finalist for the 2009 Women's Business Network Award.